AFRICAN AMERICAN HOME REMEDIES

A PRACTICAL GUIDE
WITH
USAGE AND APPLICATION DATA

3/8/18

Tom & Helen,

Best regards

thanks!,

Eddie L Boyd

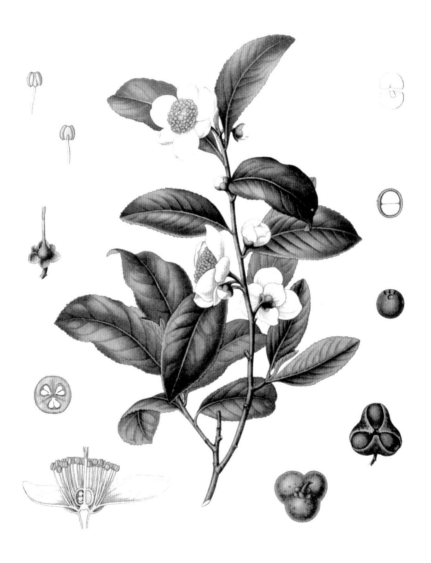

African American Home Remedies

A Practical Guide
with
Usage and Application Data

Eddie L. Boyd, Pharm. D., M.S.
Leslie A. Shimp, Pharm. D., M.S.

University of Louisiana at Lafayette Press
2014

University of Louisiana at Lafayette Press
P.O. Box 40831
Lafayette, LA 70504-0831
http://ulpress.org

Printed on acid-free paper.

Library of Congress Cataloging-in-Publication Data

Boyd, Eddie L., author.
  African American home remedies : a practical guide with usage and application data / Eddie L. Boyd and Leslie A. Shimp.
    p. ; cm.
  Includes bibliographical references.
  ISBN 978-1-935754-32-9 (alk. paper)
  I. Shimp, Leslie A., author. II. Title.
  [DNLM: 1. Medicine, African Traditional—United States. 2. African Americans—ethnology—United States. 3. Phytotherapy—methods—United States. WB 55.A3]
  RM666.H33
  615.8′808996073—dc23
    2014003524

DISCLAIMER: The information contained in this book is NOT intended to substitute for advice from a medical professional. The information is provided for educational purposes only and to provide the reader with information regarding how some African Americans used home remedies and herbal products in the past. Information regarding the demographic factors related to the use of home remedies and herbs by African Americans is also provided. The reader should NOT use the information to diagnose or treat any health problems and/or diseases without consulting with a qualified health professional. The decision to use, or not to use, any information in this book in any manner is the sole prerogative and responsibility of the reader.

I want to dedicate this book to my parents, especially to my mother, who successfully raised twelve children in a very hostile environment with absolutely no financial resources. I regret that I never told her how much I loved and respected her.

With love and respect for my mom.

Her Twelfth Child and Seventh Son,
Eddie L. Boyd

I want to dedicate this book to my parents — my mother, a nurse, demonstrated caring for the health of others and my father who started me thinking about pharmacy as a career.

In addition, I dedicate this book to the many people, some of them my patients, who discussed, inquired about, and shared information regarding the use of natural products to improve health. Thank you for the interesting conversations and for being a partner in seeking health and well-being.

Leslie A. Shimp

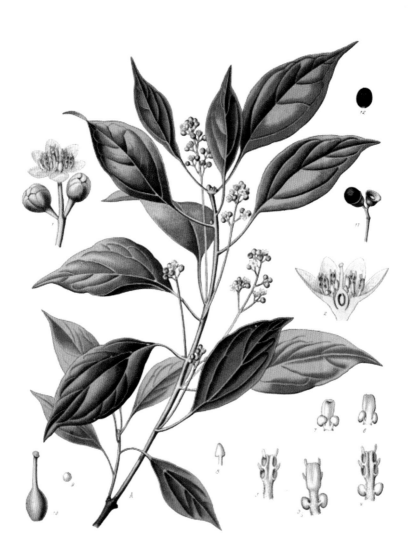

TABLE OF CONTENTS

Acknowledgments

The authors appreciate the work done by Marvie L. Hackney, who spent many hours helping organize and solicit respondents for the first Michigan study; the many interviewers who collected data for the study; Michael Reiter, who was instrumental in creating and organizing the study; and Richard L. Douglass, who helped analyze the study data.

The authors also appreciate the work done by the many University of Michigan doctor of pharmacy students who used the data from the second Michigan study to satisfy their University of Michigan College of Pharmacy required research commitments.

Additionally, the authors wish to thank Stephanie D. Taylor, Ph.D., who helped analyze the data from the second Michigan study used in this book and coauthored a publication discussing how the data supported the theoretical models.

The authors also wish to thank James S. Jackson, Ph.D., Director of the Institute of Social Research and Director of the National Survey of Black Americans, University of Michigan Survey Research Center, who granted the authors permission to conduct secondary analysis of the data.

Lastly, we want to express our deep appreciation to Jeffrey Roux who spent numerous hours reviewing and proofreading this book. He made several suggestions that were invaluable in this book's preparation.

INTRODUCTION

For a significant portion of the African American population, the use of home remedies and herbs was an important component of health care when they had no health insurance and/or no funds and were unable to regularly visit conventional health care practitioners. Some of this population continues to use these preparations today. Many of these individuals utilize both scientific and folk medicine. However, they may or may not inform their health care providers about their use of folk medicine. Some believers in folk practices and beliefs are reluctant to discuss their self-medication practices and beliefs with conventional health care providers for fear of being belittled, misunderstood, and labeled ignorant.[1] Based on the authors' experience, the use of folk medicine by African Americans frequently includes the use of both home remedies and herbs.

The authors, in conjunction with staff from the Institute of Gerontology and the Institute of Social Research at the University of Michigan, conducted two studies of the use of home remedies and herbal preparations by African Americans. In order to ensure that everyone involved with the studies was "speaking the same language," the authors looked for published definitions of herbs and home remedies. The authors could find no published definition of home remedy so the following working descriptive definition was written to ensure that interviewers and respondents were using the term in the same context.

HERB (H): any seed plant whose stem withers away to the ground after each season's growth, as distinguished from a tree or shrub whose woody stem lives from year to year; or any plant used as a medicine, seasoning, or flavoring.[2]

HOME REMEDY (HR) 1: any substance that can be purchased or obtained without a prescription and in most cases must be mixed, diluted, dried, etc. prior to use or, 2: any substance that can be purchased without a prescription and used for medical purposes in a manner not indicated on the label. Additionally, any substance that can be obtained and used for unapproved medical purposes (like cow manure and salt pork) may be considered a home remedy.

The definition of home remedy was written in 1977, long before the Office of Alternative Medicine was established in 1992 and the National Center for Complementary and Alternative Medicine (NCCAM) was established by Congress in 1998.

After NCCAM was established, complementary and alternative medicines (CAMs) were generally classified as natural products or mind and body practices. Using NCCAM terminology, most of the 163 home remedies and herbs from the Michigan studies can loosely be classified as natural products. However, using CAM terminology it is difficult to classify some of the practices, like taking a small pouch of asafetida and tying it with a string around an infant's neck to prevent colds, and/or tying a penny with a hole in it around a small child's neck to help alleviate pain associated with teething. It is also questionable where ingredients like kerosene and turpentine should be placed using CAM terminology.

Study Respondents' Descriptions of Home Remedies

All of the respondents in the first Michigan study said they either used or had personal knowledge of the remedies they discussed, and they gave a variety of answers to the question, "What does the term 'home remedy' mean to you?" The following statements are a sampling of their responses:

"Any type of remedy used at home that is grown in my own garden, or from a health food store, or that someone gives me. Some remedies are not from the doctor."

"Things you have around the house that you use for medicines."

"Roots, weeds, mullein roots, many herbs, and bark from trees."

"It's something to use without spending a lot of money."

"Things in your kitchen you can use to make you feel better."

"Types of things I take to cure ailments. We used them at home instead of going to the hospital."

"Things I learned from my parents — we did not have medicines and doctors."

Many home remedy formulas and beliefs date back to the days of slavery when most African Americans lived in poverty in rural areas of the South. As one respondent said, "When my grandmother was growing up they didn't have doctors, so home remedies were used. They worked and I have been using them ever since." Another respondent said, "My mother raised me up on them because we lived in the country. We didn't know about doctors."

Formulas for most home remedies were passed along from one generation to the next by word of mouth; 94% of the respondents reported that this was how they learned about remedies. When asked if they had any remedy recipes written down, 82% of the sample said no.

Use of Home Remedies

Two national surveys indicate that the use of home remedies is common.[3] In a 1983 survey of the U.S. population 14% of the respondents indicated they used home remedies to initially treat health problems, whereas 9% called or went to a doctor or dentist, 11% used a prescription medication available in the home, 34% used a nonprescription drug, and 30% did not treat the problem.[4] In a similar survey conducted in 1992, researchers found that 14% of the respondents reported using home remedies, 15% called or went to a doctor or dentist, 11% used a prescription already in the home, 32% used a nonprescription drug, and 28% did not treat the problem.[5] In both studies some respondents took more than one action to alleviate the problem. Although conducted on a national level, these surveys did not include a representative sample of African Americans.

Adult use of complementary and alternative medicine (CAM), including herbs, has increased substantially in the past two decades. In 2002, national estimates of CAM use by U.S. adults (including prayer) in the previous twelve months was 62.1% and it was 67.6 to 71.2% for African Americans.[6] When prayer specifically for health reasons was excluded, 36% of adults used CAM therapy during the preceding twelve months. In 2002, the most common use of CAM by the general population included deep breathing exercises, herbs, and relaxation. African Americans have a similar profile with prayer for health reasons, herbs, and relaxation as the most popular.[7] In 2007, approximately four out of ten adults had used CAM in the past twelve months, and the most commonly used therapies were non-vitamin, non-mineral, natural products (17.7%) and deep breathing (12.7%). American Indian or Alaska Native adults (50.3%) and white adults (43.1%) were more likely to use CAM than Asian adults (39.9%) or African American adults (25.5%).[8]

Three primary sources of information were used to prepare this publication—the personal experience of one of the authors (Eddie L. Boyd) and two studies conducted at the University of Michigan.[9] Prior to conducting the studies at the University of Michigan, the authors believed that home remedy and herbal use by African Americans was related to age, gender, educational level, individual or family income, religiosity, health care coverage or insurance, and contact with a grandparent or great-grandparent when growing up. The results of the studies provided the authors with new insights regarding the use of home remedies and herbal products by African Americans.

First Author's Relevant Personal Background

The first source of information is based on personal experience by one of the authors (Eddie L. Boyd). He is the twelfth of thirteen children (one child died at birth) from a very poor farm family. He grew up in Canton, Mississippi, in the 1940-50s. His family had absolutely no money to go to doctors and no health insurance. Whenever he and his siblings were ill, or as his mother would say, "she wanted to keep them from catching something," she used home remedies or herbs for their treatment.

Approximately one-half of the home remedies and herbs discussed in this publication were used by the Boyd family. Some of the most common uses of remedies by the family were for coughs, colds, and stomach problems (diarrhea and constipation) in children. In adults they were commonly used for coughs, colds, stomach problems, and muscle aches and pains. Laxatives were also commonly used in adults and children for "spring cleaning." A common misperception among some African Americans was that laxatives were useful for treatment of the common cold. Children were given laxative tablets for this purpose, and laxatives were used by some adult family members to treat liver problems.

FIRST MICHIGAN STUDY

The second source of information is from a study entitled "Home Health Care Among the Black Elderly" funded by a grant provided by the Administration on Aging, Office of Human Development Services, Department of Health, Education, and Welfare, to the Institute of Gerontology at the University of Michigan from October 1977 to September 1978. Information derived from this study was published in 1984.[10]

The goal of the interviews was to obtain concise information about the constituents of home remedies and to gain an understanding of the conditions under which the remedies were used by elderly African Americans. The specific objectives of the study were:

- To create a compendium of home remedies used by elderly African Americans;
- To determine demographic characteristics of those elderly African Americans who use home remedies;
- To examine the beliefs and perceptions which motivate elderly African Americans to seek adjuncts to "scientific" medical treatment;
- To examine methods by which information about home remedies is disseminated within the African American community; and
- To investigate changes in home remedy practices that are the result of population migration.

The project staff developed a sample design and interview protocol for the study, selected and trained eight interviewers, designed and pre-tested the 179-question, fifty-

1

seven-page interview questionnaire, designed the analysis procedures, and analyzed the data. Data was collected for the project to accomplish the previously listed objectives. The information gathered included the names of the remedies, their ingredients, and their use. The study design did not include the calculation of the incidence or prevalence of home remedy use in the African American community or any other population.

Other than the considerations of age and ethnicity, the only criteria for inclusion in the sample was the acknowledged use and advocacy of home remedies. The features of the sample were self-selection on the basis of the respondent's acknowledged use of home remedies and herbs and identification by others in the community as home remedy and herb users.

Data regarding 163 home remedies and herbs was collected. Based on the definitions discussed earlier, ninety of the products were home remedies and seventy-three were herbs. Additionally, the following information was collected: place of birth; place of residence during childhood, teen, and adult years; number of children; income; type of dwelling; religion; education; work experience; health care coverage; method of prescription payment; and satisfaction with life.

The following table contains a summary of some of the basic demographic data for the respondents:

Table 1: Basic Demographic Data

Demographic Variable	Number (Percentage) of Respondents
Sex	
Male	12 (25)
Female	38 (75)
Age (Years)	
50-64	17 (35)
65-70	19 (36)
71-85	14 (29)

Marital Status	
Single	4 (8)
Married, living with spouse	21 (42)
Married, living separately	1 (2)
Divorced	5 (10)
Widowed	19 (38)

Additionally, forty-seven of the respondents (94%) were born at home, and all but six were born in southern or border states. The respondents were born in the following states: Alabama (10); Arkansas (3); Florida (1); Georgia (7); Kentucky (2); Louisiana (4); Michigan (3); Mississippi (6); North Carolina (3); Ohio (2); South Carolina (2); Tennessee (4); Texas (1); and Canada (1). Based on 1970 census information, all of the states except Michigan and Ohio, and Canada, are located in the southern region.

When the study was conducted, all of the respondents resided in southeastern Michigan, including Ann Arbor, Detroit, Ecorse, Inkster, Sumpter Township, River Rouge, and Ypsilanti.

Most of the individuals spent their childhood in the state of their birth. The respondents were evenly divided between those who spent their childhood years in large cities, those who lived in small towns or suburbs, and those who lived on farms or in rural areas. During their teenage years most respondents remained in the South; nine spent their teenage years in Michigan. By the time the respondents had reached adulthood, forty-two (84%) were living in northern states; forty (80%) lived in Michigan.

Forty-nine out of fifty persons in the study sample were Protestant, and one respondent was Catholic. Of the Protestants, over one-half were Baptists, and about a quarter were Methodists. Nearly three-quarters of the respondents attended services or other church activities at least once a week. Only three persons said they did not go to church at all. Two-thirds of the group considered themselves very religious.

Nearly all of the respondents reported that they pray regularly, read the Bible frequently, listen to and/or watch religious programs on the radio and/or television, and participate in religious activities.

A little over half (54%) of the group had less than nine years of formal education. Twenty persons completed high school, and three continued beyond high school, studying a trade such as cosmetology, practical nursing, or carpentry.

Social Security income was the main source of financial support for 70% of the respondents. Other major sources of income were pensions from work, wages, and Supplemental Social Security income. Additionally, seven persons received some income from veterans benefits, rental property, or private retirement plans. Total yearly income was under $3,000 a year for 43% of the sample. Only four persons received more than $10,000 per year. In 1978, the average household income for whites was $40,200 and for African Americans was $24,175.[11]

Regarding health insurance, 22% of the respondents carried only private health insurance; 8% had Medicare and Medicaid in addition to private insurance; 10% had Medicare only; and 10% had Medicaid only. The remainder of the respondents had other insurance coverage or were unsure of the type of health coverage they had. For prescriptions, 42% of the respondents paid with cash and 32% used Medicaid.

Why Home Remedies Were Used

There seems to be a strong relationship between home remedy use and religious beliefs. The study sample was a highly religious group. They believed that God gave them wisdom to make remedies and created every tree, leaf, and living thing for man's use and benefit. Common remedy ingredients, for instance, were readily available in and around the respondents' homes. These included: red clay, hog hoofs, corn silk, chinaberries, camphor gum, mullein leaves, sage, turpentine, lemons, red onions, urine, baking soda, peppermint, red vinegar, sulfur, and molasses.

Several factors explain why individuals in this study were motivated to self-medicate with home remedies: 62% percent said they used home remedies basically because the remedies worked for them; 24% cited financial consideration—"It's cheaper than going to the doctor"; while another 20% said they used home remedies because the remedies worked for their parents. Others mentioned that home remedies "are better than doctors' medicine" and "cure quicker than doctors' medicine."

Other factors in respondents' decision to self-medicate were the period in their life in which they learned about home remedies and the way in which they learned. Most of the group reported learning about the uses of home remedies during early childhood. Most of the respondents were taught by their mothers and learned by watching their mother prepare concoctions when a family member was ill.

Of those interviewed, 58% said they preferred home remedies to nonprescription and prescription medicines. In comparing the effectiveness of home remedies to nonprescription and prescription medications, 52% of the respondents felt that home remedies worked better than commercially prepared drugs. Additionally, respondents felt that home remedies could prevent illnesses (56%) and "cure" or take away a problem (67%), while prescription and nonprescription medicines just made the person feel better. However, 32% believed prescription drugs could cure, and 23% thought nonprescription preparations could cure.

After seeing a doctor, 16% of the respondents said they would use home remedies if the physician did not give or prescribe a medicine for their compliant. One person said he would use a home remedy if a prescription medication he was taking had adverse effects on him; another said he would use a home remedy if the prescribed medicine was too expensive.

Respondents sometimes used home remedies in conjunction with over-the-counter drugs or prescriptions. Three people reported using home remedies with prescription medicines and six people used home remedies with nonprescription products. When asked what they depended on most to heal them, more than three-quarters of the respondents said home remedies. Only 15% depended on the doctor, 6% depended on prescription medications, and 3% relied on nonprescription preparations for healing.

Home remedies were used preventively (56%), before going to the doctor (48%), instead of seeing a doctor (14%), while being treated by a doctor (10%), or only if a prescription medicine had failed (8%). Some respondents said that whether or not they used home remedies depended on the condition or illness they had. One man stated that he used home remedies when he could not see a doctor or if he lacked the funds to go to a doctor. Several people said they used home remedies mostly in the wintertime. Others said they used home remedies as a spring tonic and during the winter months to ward off colds and other ailments.

When a home remedy was used that did not work, 60% of the sample indicated that they would go to a doctor, 8% would change ingredients, an equal percent would do nothing, 4% would seek information from other persons knowledgeable about home remedies, and 2% would change the dosage. The elderly respondents thought the persons who knew the most about home remedies were other older people like themselves. The majority (90%) of the sample felt people over the age of sixty were most knowledgeable about home remedies.

Similar numbers of respondents reported that they were asked for information on remedies "frequently," "not so frequently," and "never." Of those sampled, 21% estimated they were asked for such advice once a week, 18% said they were asked once a month, 12% said twice a month, and 24% said two or three times a year. Most persons (55%) said they were asked for information less often than they used to be. About one-third felt the frequency was about the same.

Various reasons were given by respondents to explain the decline in the frequency of requests they received for remedy information. Thirty-six percent of the sample felt nuclear families fostered less interactions and communication with members of the extended family. Twenty-four percent said people see their doctors more often. Two people felt that greater prosperity was responsible for the decline, in that people have more money to pay for the drugs doctors prescribe and Medicaid and Medicare programs made it easier for the elderly to receive a doctor's care.

All but two respondents felt that home remedy users were respected by people in the community. Most felt remedy users were respected because of the cures remedies bring. Respondents discussed remedies with friends and relatives and recommend remedies when someone was sick. Those who felt remedy users were not respected believed the lack of respect stemmed from remedies being too old fashion: "they are old fogey ideas and the remedies smell bad."

According to the survey respondents, very few health care providers inquired about home remedy use or made suggestions about continuing or stopping remedy use. Eighty percent of the respondents answered "no" to the question, "Do doctors know about the home remedies you have used?" Of the 20% who said "yes," one person said a doctor told him home remedies were harmless. Eight respondents felt nurses, pharmacists, and physicians approved of the use of home remedies. Seven doctors, two nurses, and a pharmacist were reported to indicate home remedies as useful. Two physicians were said to have told respondents that home remedies are useless. A doctor, a nurse, and a pharmacist were reported to have said that home remedies are dangerous, although no specific remedies were singled out. Only one person said a doctor told him to stop using home remedies.

The respondents themselves did not consider home remedies dangerous. There were few remedies described where it is advisable to avoid alcohol or certain foods. Most respondents seemed to use a particular remedy only with specific conditions present, and there was little evidence to suggest respondents used home remedies in a careless manner.

The majority of respondents (87%) said the recipes or formulas for home remedies have not changed over the years. The 13% who said recipes have changed attributed the changes to difficulty in obtaining ingredients.

The respondents in this study indicated that the incidence of home remedy use has changed with time. Of the persons interviewed, 72% said they used home remedies more often when they were younger, 11% said they used remedies about as often in past years as they did at the time of the study, and 13% reportedly used remedies less often. Reasons given for a decline in frequency include being under a doctor's care, respondents' taking better care of themselves and being healthier than when they were younger, and remedies no longer being tolerable to the system. Declining health was the reason given for greater current use of remedies. Slightly more than three-quarters (78%) of the respondents said people over fifty years old used more home remedies than younger people. Respondents said they themselves used home remedies as frequently as their parents did, but their children used remedies less frequently.

Just about everybody in the respondents' family knew about the use of home remedies—children, parents, aunts and uncles, and maternal and paternal grandparents. More than half (58%) of the respondents reported that they taught their children about home remedy uses. Daughters were most likely to be taught (42%), but 28% of the respondents taught their sons.

On the other hand, most respondents reported that they had not been chosen to learn the fundamentals of concocting and administering home remedies. In most instances, everyone in the family learned by watching their mother prepare remedies and by consuming or using them. Several respondents felt they learned a lot about home remedies because they were the oldest or only child in the family.

Population migration is responsible for some of the changes in home remedy practices and uses. The majority of the respondents grew up in the South, and many stated certain ingredients used in home remedies had become difficult or impossible to obtain. Thirty-five ingredients were named in response to the question, "Which of the ingredients you use or used to use are hardest to find now?" Some of the hardest-to-find ingredients were red precipitate, "devils' shoe strings," buttermilk soap, tallow, asafetida, fig juice, sassafras, calamus roots, quinine, rabbit tobacco, rock candy, and Dr. Glosser's cigarettes. Thirty-seven percent of the respondents said they patronize particular pharmacies because they carry ingredients needed to make home remedies.

Over half of the group reported having a favorite remedy. Some of the favorites included:

- Lemon and onions for chest colds
- Alcohol and vinegar for arthritis
- Salt for bowel movements
- Peppermint with red vinegar for high blood pressure
- Sage tea for bronchial and sinus conditions
- Jupiter tar, Vicks VapoRub, sulfur, and molasses for spring tonic
- Kerosene and sugar for coughs

All ethnic groups have home remedies and herbs that they have traditionally used to treat illnesses. The degree of overlap among the ingredients used by various ethnic groups is somewhat surprising. For example, there is a more than a 60% overlap between the ingredients reported by the respondents in the first Michigan study and the ingredients reported by women homesteaders in Saskatchewan between 1882 and 1914. Some of the overlapping ingredients were things like the less commonly used goose grease and gun powder.[12]

Recipes for home remedies change somewhat as remedy users migrate to parts of the country where traditional ingredients are scarce. Respondents felt the medicines made from revised formulas were not as effective as the ones to which they were accustomed.

Interview questions explored respondents' motivation to seek adjuncts to "scientific" medical treatment. Responses showed that African American believers in folk medicine turn to the professional health care provider when their own methods fail. They supplement home remedies with scientific practices because they feel neither mode is adequate independently. Persons who used home remedies generally consulted a physician for unfamiliar ailments and very serious conditions such as heart trouble or cancer.

The study described the home health care practices of a small group of people and showed that African American patients take many substances without their doctor's knowledge, despite the potential for dangerous interactions between prescribed medications and folk remedies.

Second Michigan Study

The second Michigan study was an analysis of the data from the National Survey of Black Americans (NSBA) study conducted by James S. Jackson, Ph.D., and associates at the University of Michigan Survey Research Center.[13] The analysis represented the first national look at family and individual use of home remedies and herbal products by African Americans. The NSBA study was a nationally representative cross-sectional sample of 2,107 adult (eighteen years and older) African Americans living in the continental United States in 1979 and 1980. National multistage probability sampling was used. The sample was self-weighting and every African American household in the continental United States had an equal probability of being selected. A 118-page, 342-question instrument was used to conduct in-home surveys. The data was collected in 1979 and 1980 and analyzed in 1995-99. The results were published in 2000.[14]

Many of the herbs and home remedies obtained in the first Michigan study were mentioned by the 1,439 respondents in the NBSA study who responded positively to the question, "Did your family ever use any home remedies to cure illnesses when you were growing up?" The purpose of the second Michigan study was to examine home remedy and herbal use by African American individuals and their families and assess the relationship between socio-demographic characteristics and home remedy and herbal use. Prior to analysis of the data and based on the results of the first Michigan study, previously published reports regarding home remedy and herbal use by African Americans, and the authors' experience, Figures 1 and

2 were developed as models of the theoretical relationships expected between the respondents' family and the respondents' home remedy and herbal use and socio-demographic variables. After the models were developed, the data was analyzed to determine if the theoretical models were supported.

Figure 1: Family Use of Home Remedies Model

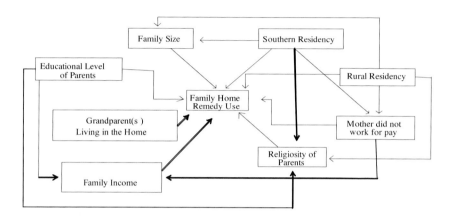

Figure 2: Individual Use of Home Remedies Model

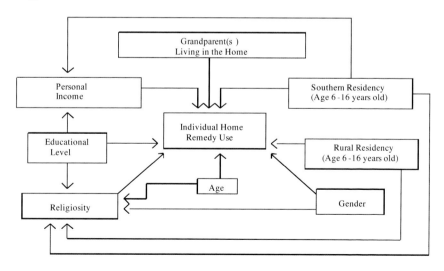

The anticipated relationships by the respondents' families are indicated in Figure 1. We expected to find that the educational level of the parents and importance of religion to the family were related to family home remedy use. We also expected rural residency, family size, and whether or not the mother worked for pay to have some influence on home remedy use. These factors may affect socioeconomic status of the family and the ability to pay for health care services. Additionally, southern residency was expected to affect family home remedy use. Studies have shown that African Americans who were born in the South are more likely to use home remedies.[15]

A grandparent residing in the home while the respondents were growing up was expected to influence the family's use of home remedies. Previous research supports the assumption that information about home remedy use is passed on by word of mouth and may be related to living with a grandparent.[16] Earlier studies indicate that the use of home remedies by families is associated with the decreased educational level of the parents[17] and increased importance of religion.[18] Region of residency has previously been found to be positively associated with family home remedy use.[19] It has been reported previously that rural residency is positively associated with family use of home remedies.[20] An association between family size and home remedy use has not been previously reported but was added to the model because the authors postulated that it may be related to decreased socioeconomic status of the family, decreased access to the organized health care system, and increased use of home remedies.

We expected to find that individual home remedy use was related to lower educational level, which may influence personal income and importance of religion, and personal income may be influenced by southern residency. The assumption that individual home remedy users were more likely to have a lower educational level had been supported by previous research.[21] The authors hypothesized that importance of religion may have a direct effect on individual home remedy use and importance of religion may be influenced by age, gender, and by rural and southern residency, especially early childhood residency. The authors also hypothesized that individual home remedy use was influenced by an elderly relative (e.g., a grandparent) residing in the home while the child was growing up. Previous research showed that information about home remedy use was passed on by word of mouth, frequently to female family members.[22]

Earlier reports indicate that individual home remedy use is positively associated with decreased socioeconomic status.[23] However, more recent research found that this trend may also be changing in regard to the use of home remedies and other alternative therapy.[24] These studies report that individual users of alternative or unconventional therapies are more likely to be educated and have higher than average incomes. Expectations of gender differences in home remedy use are consistent with previous work indicating that women are frequently the family caregivers and the healing role is passed from mother to daughter.[25] Previous research has found that individual home remedy users were often older adults.[26] However, there is no strong empirical support for the older user theory. In a study by Stewart, the average age of people who visited African American healers was fifty-one years.[27] Moreover, Banahan and Frate found that home remedy use was not related to age.[28]

The data were coded using the 1970 U.S. Census designations of dividing the United States into four regions: North East, North Central, South, and West. Formatting of the question regarding individual home remedy use made the answer to the question dependent on a positive response to the question "Did your family use any home remedies to cure illness while you were growing up?" Respondents whose families did not use home remedies while they were growing up may have been using home remedies when the survey was done, and their use would have been missed, leading to under reporting for individuals.

The following variables were used in the data analysis:

Table 2: Variables Used in the Analysis of the Family and Individual Home Remedy Use Data

Dependent Variable	Independent Variables
Family Home Remedy Use	Family Income Family size Mother's educational level Father's educational level Importance of religion Living with a grandparent Rural residency Mother worked for pay Geographic region
Individual Home Remedy Use	Age Gender Educational level Living with a grandparent Personal income Importance of religion Rural residency Geographic region

First bivariate analysis of the independent variables with the dependent variable was conducted using logistical regression. Independent variables displaying an insignificant association with the dependent variable were eliminated from further analysis. Second, multivariate analysis was conducted to explain home remedy and herbal use as a function of all of the significant variables.

In the sample of the respondents who answered the question regarding home remedy usage, 69.6% reported that their families used home remedies, and 35.4% reported that they individually used home remedies. The demographic data for the respondents is shown in Table 3.

Table 3: Demographics Of Respondents – Second Michigan Study

Demographic Variable	Number (Percentage) of Respondents
Age (years)	
18 - 29	629 (29.6)
30 - 39	433 (20.4)
40 - 54	470 (22.1)
55 - 64	251 (11.8)
65 - 74	230 (10.8)
75 - 84	100 (4.7)
85+	12 (0.6)
Gender	
Male	797 (37.8)
Female	1,310 (62.2)
Educational level	
0-11 years	919 (46.3)
High school diploma	650 (30.8)
Some college	334 (15.9)
College degree	184 (8.7)
Personal income (dollars)	
$0-4,999	839 (39.8)
$5,000-9,999	501 (23.8)
$10,000-19,999	417 (19.8)
$20,000+	129 (6.1)
Marital status	
Married	866 (41.1)
Divorced	245 (11.6)
Separated	207 (9.8)
Widowed	305 (14.5)
Never Married	467 (22.2)
Common law	11 (0.5)

Geographic region	
North East	391 (18.6)
North Central	467 (22.2)
South	1,125 (53.4)
West	124 (5.9)
Rural residency	
Non-rural	1,665 (79.0)
Rural	442 (21.0)

As indicated in the table, 29.6% of the 2,107 respondents were less than thirty years of age, and 16.1% were sixty-five years of age or over. Only 37.8% of the sample were men. With regards to education almost one-half of the respondents (46.3%) had less than a high school education, whereas 8.7% graduated from college. Approximately 40% of the respondents reported an income of less than $5,000, and only 6.1% reported an individual income over $20,000 (based on 1978 dollars). The most prevalent marital status was married (41.1%). Over one-half of the respondents were southern residents (53.4%), and few (5.9%) resided in the West. Approximately eight out of ten (79%) respondents resided in urban areas.

Multivariate analysis indicated that family home remedy and herbal use was associated with:
- parents' educational level
- increased importance of religion
- living with a grandparent when less than sixteen years of age
- rural residence when less than sixteen years of age
- region of residency

Table 4: Significant Independent Variables Used in the Second Michigan Study (Family Home Remedy and Herbal Use)

Independent Variable	Comment
Parents educational level	Mother's education and father's education were significantly associated with families' use of home remedies. More specifically, families where the father had eleven years or less of education were 77% more likely to use home remedies than families where the father had some college or a college degree.
Importance of religion	Individuals who reported religion as being only fairly important or not too important to their families were 38.3% and 53.3% less likely to report that their families used home remedies than were individuals who reported that religion was very important to them.
Living with a grandparent when less than sixteen years of age	Individuals not living with a grandparent while growing up were 37.9% less likely to report that their families used home remedies than those individuals who lived with their grandparents while growing up.
Rural residence when less than sixteen years of age	Those individuals who reported living in a non-rural area were 28.5% less likely to report that their families used home remedies than individuals living in a rural area.
Region of residency	The South and the North Central regions were especially associated with family home remedy use. Many African Americans migrated to the North Central region from the South.

The effect of each significant independent variable was determined by multivariate analysis for its effect on individual home remedy and herbal use. Variables having an effect on individual home remedy use were:
- age
- gender
- educational level
- living with a grandparent when less than sixteen years of age
- region of residency

Table 5: Significant Independent Variables Used in the Analysis of the Individual Home Remedy and Herbal Use Data

Independent Variable	Comment
Age	Younger individuals were more likely to use home remedies and herbal products than were older individuals.
Gender	Males were 47.4% less likely to use home remedies than females.
Educational level	Individuals with a high level of education were more likely to use home remedies and herbal products than individuals with less education.
Living with a grandparent when less than sixteen years of age	Individuals not living with a grandparent as a child were 26.3% less likely to use home remedies than individuals living with a grandparent as a child.
Region of residency	Individuals residing in the South and North Central regions were more likely to report the use of home remedies than individuals residing in the North East or West. High usage in the North Central region was partially a result of migration to the large cities in this region by African Americans from the South.

Limitations Regarding Use of Study Data

Because the primary focus of the NSBA study was not home remedy use, some of the data regarding the variables used to determine home remedy use are missing. Clearly, the disadvantage of data collected from both Michigan studies is their age, and much has changed over time. However, analysis of the data from this study allowed the authors to determine the demographic variables related to family and individual home and herbal use of African Americans. This analysis is important because self-care, increased marketing, and use of herbal products have increased dramatically in the past three decades. Consumers need as much factual information as possible about these products and their use.

Conditions Treated with Home Remedies and Herbs

(The conditions and treatments listed are those that were indicated by the fifty study respondents from the first Michigan study.)

CONDITION	TREATMENT
Abortion	Black Pepper, Quinine, Turpentine, Vinegar
Abscess	Egg (skin), Epsom Salt, Flaxseed Tea, Lard, Salt,
Acne	Camphor, Egg (skin), Petroleum Jelly, Turpentine, Witch Hazel
Alcoholism	Flour
Anemia	Blackberry Root, Black Draught, Sage Tea, Sassafras, Steak (beef), Sulfur, Whiskey
Arthritis	Alcohol, Alfalfa Tea, Ammonia, Apple Cider, Camphor, Castor Oil, Celery Leaf Tea, Coffee, Cucumber, Dandelion, Egg (white), Fat Meat (grease), Gasoline, Kerosene, Lard, Lemon Juice, Mothballs, Olive Oil, Parsley Tea, Pine Needles, Turpentine, Vinegar

Asthma	Asafetida, Blood (cow), Camphor, Cedarwood Oil, Coltsfoot Tea, Eucalyptus Oil, Glycerin, Honey, Jimson Weed, Pine Needles, Saltpeter, Sugar, Sulfur, Vicks VapoRub, Whiskey, Tea
Athlete's foot	Bleach, Epsom Salt, Roman Cleanser
Back Pain	Alfalfa, Corn Silk Tea, Red Clover Tea, Salt,
Bad Breath	Baking Soda, Calamus, Cardamom Seed, Catnip, Pine Needle Tea
Baldness	Chinaberry Root Tea
Bedsores	Buckthorn, Sugar
Bedwetting	Pine Needle Tea
Belching	Baking Soda, Cola
Black Eye	Apple, Apple Cider, Leeches, Liver (raw), Potatoes, Salt, Steak (beef), Witch Hazel
Blackouts	Ammonia
Blurred Vision	Garlic
Boils	Buckthorn, Egg (skin), Fat Meat, Milkweed, Turpentine
Bronchitis	Asafetida, Honey, Lard, Pine Needle Tea, Vicks VapoRub

Bruises	Camphor, Epsom Salt, Iron
Bunions	Roman Cleanser
Burns	Aloe Vera, Baking Soda, Butter, Devil's Dust, Lard, Petroleum Jelly, Onion Juice
Burning on Urination	Sweet Spirit of Nitre
Cataracts	Coffee, Coconut Milk
Chest Pain	Asafetida, Baking Soda, Calamus, Black Pepper, Peppermint, Spearmint, Vinegar
Chills	Black Pepper, Lemon Juice, Mullein, Peach Leaves, Quinine, Ragweed, Sunflower
Colds	Asafetida, Black Draught, Garlic, Honey, Horehound, Juniper, Kerosene, Lemon Juice, Molasses, Mullein, Onion, Sage Tea, Sassafras, Sugar (rock candy), Turpentine, Vinegar, Whiskey
Cold in the Eye	Boric Acid, Epsom Salt, Molasses, Salt, Tea, Witch Hazel
Cold Sores	Alum, Camphor, Earwax, Fat Meat, Kerosene, Salt, Sulfur, Turpentine, Petroleum Jelly, Vicks VapoRub
Corns/Calluses	Alcohol, Epson Salt, Onion, Roman Cleanser, Turpentine, Vinegar

Constipation	Blackberry Root, Buckthorn, Celery Leaf Tea, Lemon Juice, Mustard, Senna Leaves, Turnip (garden), Whiskey
Convulsions-Epilepsy	Mustard
Cramps	Buttermilk, Calamus, Camphor, Flour, Ginger, Nutmeg, Paregoric, Pennyroyal, Sugar (Rock Candy), Tea, Turpentine, Whiskey
Cuts*	Axle Grease, Kerosene, Milkweeds, Petroleum Jelly, Salt, Soot, Sulfur, Vitamin E
Denture Problems-Toughen Gums	Alum, Baking Soda, Mercurochrome
Diabetes Mellitus	Blackberry Leaf, Cucumber, Dandelion, Huckleberry Leaf, Lemon, Peanuts (raw), Sage Tea
Diarrhea	Blackberry Root, Black Pepper, Flour, Grape Juice, Peach Bark, Raspberry
Dizziness	Aspirin, Black Draught, Epsom Salt, Peppermint
Dropsy	Cedarwood Oil, Celery Leaf Tea, Epsom Salt, Holly Bark, Lard
Dry Skin	Olive Oil, Petroleum Jelly
Earache	Betsy Bug, Molasses, Olive Oil,

	Rabbit Tobacco, Syrup, Tobacco (smoke), Urine (male)
Edema	Brown Paper Bag, Corn Silk Tea, Epsom Salt, Iron, Mullein, Vinegar
Fainting	Ammonia
Feeling Poorly	Dandelion Leaves
Feminine Cleansing	Vinegar, Witch Hazel
Fever	Alcohol, Baking Soda, Black Draught, Camphor, Common Christian Leaves, Cow Manure, Fat Meat (grease), Lemon, Mullein, Onion, Salt, Sweet Oil, Vicks VapoRub
Fever Blister	Alum, Baking Soda, Buckthorn, Camphor, Earwax, Kerosene, Petroleum Jelly, Salt, Turpentine, Vicks VapoRub
Foul Smelling Urine	Buckthorn
Frostbite	Castor Oil, Fat Meat (grease), Lard, Pine, Quinine, Salt, Turnip (roasted), Turpentine
Gas	Asafetida, Baking Soda, Calamus, Chamomile, Epsom Salt, Garlic, Vinegar
Glaucoma	Coffee

Goiter	Iodine, Salt
Hair Loss	Chinaberry Root Tea, Coon Fat, Egg (whole), Iodine, Petroleum Jelly, Quinine, Red Precipitate, Sage Tea, Sulfur, Sweet Oil, Whiskey
Hay Fever	Aspirin, Rabbit Tobacco, Sage Tea, Salt
Headaches	Brown Paper Bag, Camphor, Epsom Salt, Jimson Weed, Lemon, Milk of Magnesia, Peppermint, Potatoes, Quinine, Vicks VapoRub, Vinegar, Whiskey
Hearing Loss	Camphor
Heartburn	Black Pepper, Calamus, Chamomile, Cola, Rhubarb, Sugar, Vinegar
Heart Trouble	Asafetida
Hemorrhoids	Butter, Flour, Kerosene, Lard, Olive Oil, Sage Tea, Turpentine, Vicks VapoRub,
Hernia	Castor Oil, Milk, Sage Tea
Hiccoughs	Baking Soda
High Blood Pressure	Celery Leaf Tea, Cream of Tartar, Epsom Salt, Garlic, Lemon, Potatoes, Vinegar

Hoarseness	Alum, Baking Soda, Honey, Horehound, Iodine, Lemon, Mouthwash, Salt, Sugar, Turpentine, Vinegar
Hot Flashes	Sage Tea
Impotence	Vitamin E Oil
Infections	Epsom Salt, Fenugreek (leg ulcer infections-sugar)
Influenza	Asafetida, Baking Soda, Green Grass Tea, Honey, Hog Hoof Tea, Pine
Ingrown Toenails	Vitamin E
Insect Bites	Camphor, Salt, Snuff, Tobacco, Turpentine, Petroleum Jelly
Insomnia	Hot Milk, Nutmeg
Irregular Periods	Ginger
Jaundice	Lemon, Walnut
Kidney Problems	Celery Leaf Tea, Iodine, Lemon, Olive Oil, Sweet Spirit of Nitre, Watermelon Seed Tea
Lack of Vaginal Lubrication	Petroleum Jelly
Lice	Sulfur, Turpentine
Loss of Appetite	Asafetida, Sweet Pickles,

	(Cucumber), Thiamine
Low Blood Pressure	Iron
Malaria	Lemon
Menopause	Cohosh, Licorice
Menstrual Cramps	Camphor, Cohosh, Corn Silk Tea, Ginseng, Licorice, Pennyroyal, Pepper, Sage Tea, Turpentine, Vinegar
Miscarriages	Quinine
Mouth Ulcers	Boric Acid, Mouthwash, Salt
Muscle Aches	Ammonia, Camphor, Ginger, Olive Oil, Tea, Turpentine
Nausea	Calamus, Flour, Ginger, Lemon, Peppermint, Sugar, Vinegar
Nasal Congestion	Camphor, Flour, Mustard, Peppermint, Salt
Nervousness	Catnip, Kerosene, Quinine, Sugar
Nosebleeds	Brown Paper Bag, Salt
Numbness	Olive Oil
Nursing Mothers with Inadequate Milk Production	Tea

Penile Discharge	Buckthorn
Pinkeye	Boric Acid, Egg, Epsom Salt
Pneumonia	Black Draught, Castor Oil, Fat Meat, Hog Hoof Tea, Honey, Jimson Weed, Kerosene, Lard, Lemon Juice, Lye Soap, Milk, Mullein, Olive Oil, Onion, Sage Tea, Salt, Turpentine, Vicks VapoRub, Whiskey
Poison Ivy	Gun Shell Powder, Jimson Weed, Petroleum Jelly, Sulfur, Watermelon (rind), Witch Hazel
Rashes	Baking Soda, Buckthorn, Corn Starch, Epsom Salt, Jimson Weed
Ringworms	Alcohol, Brown Paper Bag, Buckthorn, Calf Slobber, Chinaberry Root Tea, Milk, Petroleum Jelly, Shoe Polish
Runny Nose	Salt
Scabies	Lard, Sulfur
Shortness of Breath	Asafetida
Snakebites	Chicken (live), Kerosene, Turpentine
Sneezing	Camphor
Sore Throat	Alum, Baking Soda, Egg (whole), Fig Juice, Mouthwash, Olive Oil,

	Pepper (red), Salt, Syrup, Turnip, Turpentine, Urine (male), Vinegar, Whiskey
Sprains	Bittersweet, Vinegar
Sties	Alum, Quinine, Sulfate of Zinc, Tea
Tender Breasts	Alum
Thrush	Bleach, Bluing, Boric Acid, Camphor, Catnip, Petroleum Jelly, Red Alder, Salt, Sardine Oil, Whiskey
Tired Eyes	Boric Acid, Epsom Salt, Eyebright, Flaxseed Tea, Milk, Molasses, Salt, Sugar, Witch Hazel
Tiredness	Senna Leaves, Thoroughwort
Too Much Milk (While Nursing)	Camphor
Tonic	Pokeweed
Toothaches	Calamus, Camphor, Kerosene, Mouthwash, Perfume, Sloan's Liniment, Sugar, Vanilla Flavoring
To Stop Bleeding	Salt, Spider Webs, Snuff
Tuberculosis	Asafetida, Honey, Pine Needle Tea

Ulcers	Boric Acid, Flaxseed Tea, Milk
Vaginal Discharge	Baking Soda, Salt, Turpentine, Vinegar, Vicks VapoRub, Watermelon Seeds
Venereal Disease	Blackberry Root, Corn (meal), Dogwood, Egg (shell and white), Flour, Huckleberry Root, Red Shank, Sarsaparilla
Vomiting	Aspirin, Basil, Bread (burnt), Camphor, Castor Oil, Catnip, Cola, Duckweed, Lemon, Milk of Magnesia, Sugar
Warts	Buckthorn
Worms	Asafetida, Calamus, Garlic, Potatoes, Sugar, Turpentine

*Axle Grease and Kerosene were used to treat wounds when access to infection control was non-existent. Injuries frequently occurred when farm laborers were working in cotton, corn, or cane fields, and many of the laborers had no access to hot and cold running water. If the injury occurred close to a farm house, it took at least an hour to build a fire and boil contaminated water from the open cisterns used by many of the farm laborers to drink, clean wounds, and bathe.

HOME REMEDIES AND HERBS USED BY THE RESPONDENTS AND THEIR KNOWN USES

The home remedies and herbs that will be discussed are those identified in the study "Home Health Care among the Black Elderly," sponsored by the Institute of Gerontology, the University of Michigan, and funded through Grant No. 90-A129(01), from the Administration on Aging, Office of Human Development Services, United States Department of Health and Human Services. For each home remedy discussed we will include what it is used to treat, how it is used, its effectiveness, if known, and toxicities or other precautions associated with use of the product, and one of the author's (Eddie L. Boyd) experience with using the remedy. The statement that "no published scientific or clinical information or studies were found to support the use of this product" is made after approximate thirty years of monitoring the medical literature for research and teaching purposes and finding no supporting reliable clinical or scientific data. This does not mean that the herb or home remedy has no therapeutic value. It means that, thus far, based on normal scientific criteria, no studies or information attesting to its therapeutic value has been published. Many research studies are conducted and the results published because of the profits earned with patented drugs or devices. Most of the home remedies and herbs used by the respondents have little or no profit value, and therefore research with them is not regularly conducted. The uses of the herbs and remedies are those indicated by the respondents and MAY or MAY NOT be VALID and/or SAFE.

Based on the definitions discussed previously, each home remedy or herb will be identified with an (HR) or (H) following its name.

ALCOHOL (ISOPROPYL) (HR)

Study respondents used isopropyl alcohol to treat corns, calluses, insect bites, ringworms, arthritis, and fever. When applied externally, isopropyl alcohol has astringent properties. For this reason, it is used in the preparation of many prescription and nonprescription products, including insect bite, acne, hair, and hand preparations. It is used in aftershave lotions and liniments and also has been used topically for many years to treat muscle aches and pain. In fact, some isopropyl alcohol preparations are labeled "Rubbing Alcohol." It was labeled this way in many older pharmaceutical references.[29] When applied topically alcohol cools the skin as it evaporates. It has been used in this manner to reduce fever. When alcohol is applied topically over large areas of an infant's body, toxicity can occur. Isopropyl alcohol has central nervous system depressive properties and is toxic when used internally. The lethal dose by mouth is reported to be about 250 ml (approximately 8 ounces) and toxic symptoms may be produced by as little as 20 ml (approximately 1 tablespoonful).[30]

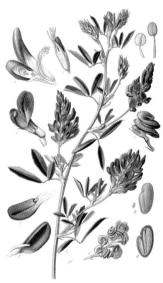

ALFALFA (H)
(MEDICAGO SATIVA, LUCERNE)

Study participants reportedly used alfalfa for the treatment of back pain and arthritis. Alfalfa has been used as a diuretic for kidney conditions and for prostate and bladder conditions. It has also been used for asthma, diabetes, arthritis, and increased cholesterol levels; however, some of the supporting studies were conducted in animals.[31] Its use as a diuretic and for kidney conditions explains why it was used by our study participants for back pain. Consumption of alfalfa leaves is relatively safe, and consumption of the seeds has been used to reduce low density proteins in individuals with type II high cholesterol.[32] However, high consumption of excessive amounts of alfalfa seeds on a long-term basis has been associated with a pronounced reduction in red blood cells, white blood cells, and platelets.[33] Consumption of alfalfa seeds has also caused the induction of lupus.[34] Alfalfa has also been used as a source of vitamin K; however, its use can antagonize the effects of anticoagulants, including warfarin.[35]

ALOE VERA (H)
(SEVERAL SYNONYMS)

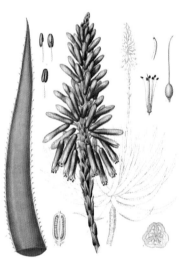

Aloe vera was reportedly used to treat burns by the study participants. It is used by rubbing a broken or cut part of the plant on the injury. Topically, aloe vera is used to treat burns, superficial wounds, psoriasis, sunburn, frostbite, inflammation, osteoarthritis, and cold sores. As an antiseptic and as a moisturizer it is also used topically. For most of these uses, aloe vera is relatively safe and effective,[36] however, some cases of allergic dermatitis have occurred after its topical use.[37] In an earlier study, applying aloe extract 0.5 percent cream topically three times daily for four weeks significantly improved and increased the resolution of psoriatic plaques compared to a placebo;[38] however, follow-up studies did not support these findings.[39] Orally, aloe vera has been used to treat osteoarthritis, inflammatory bowel disease, fever, and itching. It also has been used as a laxative. The active ingredients in the plant are a latex and gel. The gel is contained in cells in the center of the leaf and the latex in the cells adjacent to the skin of the plant. The anthraquinone laxatives contained in the latex of aloe vera can prevent water and electrolyte reabsorption.[40] Because of the strong laxative property of the latex, in 2002, FDA removed aloe from the list of active ingredients allowed to be included in nonprescription drugs marketed in the United States. Because of potential adverse effects from the oral use of the intact aloe plant or the latex, the authors recommend that they not be used, especially in children less than twelve years of age, unless recommended by a physician.

ALUM (HR)
(POTASSIUM ALUMINUM SULFATE)

Alum was used to treat sties, cold sores, fever blisters, thrush, denture problems, sore throat, hoarseness, and tender breast. Alum precipitates proteins and is a powerful astringent. This action will reduce the loss of fluids when applied to open wounds. It is used in the preparations of mouthwashes and/ or gargles and in dermatological products. Prolonged use of mouthwashes or gargles containing alum is not desirable because it may have adverse effects on teeth. Either solid alum or alum solutions have been used to stop the bleeding of superficial cuts and abrasions.[41] Excessive sweating is sometimes treated by bathing the affected parts in a mild alum solution. Stronger solutions harden the epidermis and have been used to treat soft corns and sore feet. Mixtures of alum and purified talc have been used for foot odor.

AMMONIA (HR)

Ammonia was used to treat insect bites, muscle aches, arthritis, blackouts, and fainting. Dilute ammonia solutions have been used as reflex stimulants either as smelling salts or for oral administration. Applied externally, it is used to neutralize insect stings and as a counterirritant. A dilute solution of ammonia produces redness in individuals with a light complexion and feelings of warmth when applied to the skin.[42]

Apple (H)
(*Malus domestica*, other synonyms)

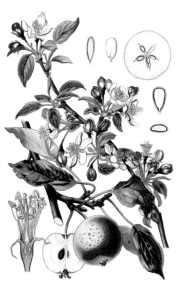

Study respondents reportedly used apple/apple cider to treat black eyes and arthritis. Apple has been used in the treatment of cancer, diabetes, dysentery, fever, heart problems, scurvy, and warts.[43] Apple has also been used in the treatment of constipation or diarrhea and the collection of gallstones.[44] Apples contain pectin, which is useful in the treatment of diarrhea and constipation. Pectin absorbs fluids from the GI tract and swells to produce bulky stools in constipation or aid in producing formed stools when an individual has diarrhea. Prior to the 1980s, Kaopectate contained kaolin (a clay) as an absorbent and pectin as an emollient. In 2004, the active ingredient in Kaopectate sold in the United States was changed to bismuth subsalicylate.

It has been reported that individuals who consume large amounts of unsweetened apple cider have a low incidence of kidney stones, gout, and rheumatism. This effect has been attributed to the diuretic effect of malic and lactic acids that may help to eliminate uric acid from the body.

The consumption of large amounts of apple seeds can lead to cyanide poisoning.[45]

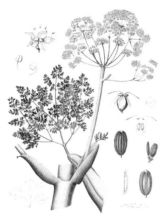

ASAFETIDA (H)
(*FERULA ASAFETIDA*, OR OTHER FERULA SPECIES, DEVIL'S DUNG)

Asafetida is a foul smelling oleo-resin. Its smell has lead to it being referred to as "Devil's Dung." It has the foul smelling odor when raw, but when it is used as a spice in cooking it delivers a flavor reminiscent of leeks. Our study respondents reportedly used it to treat chest pain, heart trouble, asthma, bronchitis, shortness of breath, tuberculosis, cold, influenza, loss of appetite, gas, and worms. Limited medical research indicates that it may be useful in the treatment of flatulence, asthma, bronchitis, and whooping cough.[46] A traditional folk remedy used by African Americans for colds in children was to place the resin in a small pouch and hang it around the child's neck. It may have worked because the foul smell prevented close encounters with individuals, including those with contagious diseases. Recent research indicates that it may produce antiviral compounds that kill the swine flu virus, H1N1.[47] The authors found little or no published clinical or scientific evidence to support the other uses listed above.

ASPIRIN (HR)
(ACETYLSALICYLIC ACID)

Study respondents reportedly used aspirin to treat dizziness, hay fever, and vomiting. Studies support the use of aspirin to treat several types of pain, to lower increased body temperature, and to decrease the risk of heart attacks. Its use for the other ailments listed has not been supported by scientific or clinical studies. Aspirin should not be used in young children because of the risk of Reyes Syndrome.

Axle Grease (HR)

Axle grease reportedly was used to treat cuts and insect bites. Traditionally, axle grease has been used to increase healing of sores and prevent infections. Axle grease originally was made of animal fats mixed with soaps or other thickening agents. Since 1859 axle grease has been made from petroleum products with soaps added. As far back as 1400 B.C., mutton fat and beef tallow were used on chariot axles to reduce friction in order to allow more speed and to slow down wear. Axle grease has been used for many years for this purpose. Lime was usually added to these fats to make their lubricating properties last longer. A well-performing axle grease typically had a high initial viscosity that decreased when shear was applied (the wheel turns on the axle). Thickening agents like tar or graphite are normally added to fatty oil based greases to increase their durability. The axle grease used by the author's (Eddie L. Boyd) family had the consistency of petroleum jelly with a dark grey or black color and was a petroleum derivative. The authors found no published clinical or scientific studies that support the use of axle grease for medical purposes.

Baking Soda (HR)
(Sodium Bicarbonate)

Baking soda was used to treat fever blisters, thrush, denture problems, bad breath, sore throat, hoarseness, chest pain, influenza, nausea, hiccoughs, belching, gas, vaginal discharge, rash, burns, and fever. Baking soda has been applied topically to treat insect bites, dermatitis, urticaria, and eczema. Topical applications of very dilute solutions can effectively be used to decrease nasal congestion. It has been used for many years as an effective antacid for minor stomach problems. Prior to the FDA's review of all of the antacids on the U.S. market, many commercial antacids contained sodium bicarbonate as the active ingredient. After the FDA review, antacid manufacturers were required to replace the sodium bicarbonate with either calcium carbonate or magnesium carbonate. FDA anticipated that the sodium ion in the bicarbonate antacids might have an adverse effect on consumers with cardiovascular problems. Baking soda has long been used as a tooth powder and it is the effective active ingredient in several commercial dentifrices. The collective results from five clinical studies on over 270 subjects demonstrated that baking soda dentifrices enhanced plaque removal effectiveness of tooth brushing to a significantly greater extent than the non-baking soda dentifrice products.[48] Sodium bicarbonate sitz baths may provide some relief of vulva irritation associated with candidal vaginal infections.[49]

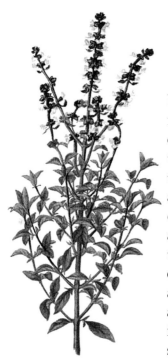

BASIL (H)
(*OCIMUM BASILICUM*)

Study respondents reportedly used basil to stop vomiting. Orally, basil is used for stomach spasms, kidney conditions, before and after childbirth to promote blood circulation, and to treat snakebites. It is also used orally as an appetite stimulant, antiflatulent, diuretic, lactation stimulant, and gargle and mouth astringent. Reportedly the health benefits of compounds contained in basil oil have potent antioxidant, anticancer, antiviral, and antimicrobial properties.[50] In India, it has been used to treat diabetes, stress, and asthma. The essential oil of basil may have antifungal and insect repellant activities.[51] Published documentation of the effectiveness for the other listed uses cannot be substantiated.

Beef Gall (Bile) (HR)

Study respondents reported that beef gall could be used to treat cuts. Reportedly beef gall has a mild laxative effect and has been used for indigestion or upset stomach. The authors found no published clinical or scientific studies that support the use of beef gall for medical purposes.

Betsy Bug (HR)
(Passalidae—Many Species)

Betsy bugs were reportedly used to treat earache. The body of the Betsy bug is broken apart between the thorax and abdomen, squeezed, and one or two drops of the body fluids are inserted into each ear to alleviate earache. The authors found no published clinical or scientific studies that support the use of Betsy bugs for medical purposes.

Bittersweet (H)
(Solanum Dulcamara, Deadly Nightshade)

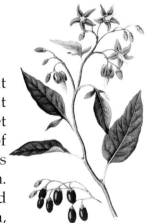

Study respondents reported that bittersweet can be used to treat sprains. The FDA classifies bittersweet as an unsafe poisonous herb because of the presence of the toxic compounds solanine, solanidine, and dulcamarin. Topically, bittersweet has been used to treat acne, skin abrasions, eczema, furuncles, and warts. It is also thought to have analgesic, anti-rheumatic, anti-inflammatory, diuretic, and sedative properties that may be related to the plant's toxicity. It is now known that all parts of this plant are poisonous,[52] and the ingestion of unripe berries can cause poisoning in children.[53] **Because of its toxicity, bittersweet should not be used for medical purposes.[54]**

BLACK DRAUGHT (H)
(SENNA—SEVERAL SPECIES: *SENNA ALEXANDRINA,* OTHER SYNONYMS)

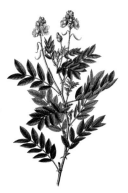

Study respondents reported that Black Draught can be used to treat dizziness, pneumonia, colds, anemia, and fever. The active ingredient in Black Draught is senna, which is a stimulant laxative.[55] Senna is an FDA approved laxative that should only be used short term in the recommended dose for the treatment of constipation. The reason that a laxative was used to treat colds, fever, pneumonia, and many other ailments was because it was commonly believed by some older African Americans that a bowel movement everyday was necessary for good health. Whenever one did not feel well, taking a laxative was the first line of therapy. In fact, Ex-Lax tablets that contained senna were referred to as "Ex-Lax Cold Tablets." The authors found no published clinical or scientific studies that support the use of senna for any of the ailments reported by the respondents.

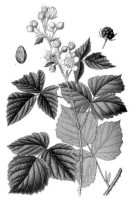

BLACKBERRY (H)
(*RUBUS*—SEVERAL SPECIES)

Study respondents used blackberry root tea to treat diarrhea and constipation. They used blackberry wine to treat anemia and venereal disease. People have used blackberries orally to treat diarrhea, edema, diabetes, gout, inflammation, and to prevent cancer and heart disease. Recent research indicates that blackberry extract has potent antioxidant, anti-proliferative, and anti-inflammatory activities.[56] It may be useful in the treatment of cancer and other inflammatory diseases.

BLEACH (HR)
(CHLORIDE OF LIME, CALCIUM HYPOCHLORITE)

Bleach was reportedly used to treat thrush and athlete's foot problems. Bleach is used as a disinfectant and antiseptic and has been used to clean the needles used by HIV positive patients. Dilute solutions (approximately 0.5%) have been used to treat minor wounds but are of questionable value when used in this manner. Dilute bleach solutions have also been used to treat toenail fungal infections but are also of questionable value when used in this manner. The FDA recently warned consumers regarding the use of a commercial product with broad health claims. The product contained 28% bleach.[57] **Bleach and bleach products should not be used for medical purposes.**

BLUEBERRY (H)
(*VACCINIUM CORYMBOSUM*)

Study respondents reported that blueberry leaves could be used for diabetes. Blueberry leaves have been used for diarrhea. Tea made from the leaves of blueberries has also been used for sore throat. Blueberries are among the fruits with the highest antioxidant properties. Recent research indicates that chemicals in blueberries may improve insulin sensitivity in obese, insulin resistant men and women.[58] Another study suggests that a dietary supplement containing sea buckthorn and blueberries may have a beneficial effect on the treatment of type 1 diabetes in children.[59] Growing evidence from tissue cultures, animal, and clinical models indicate that the fruits from blueberries and cranberries have the potential ability to limit the development and severity of certain cancers and vascular diseases, including atherosclerosis, ischemic stroke, and neurodegenerative diseases of aging.[60] Limited research also suggests that blueberry supplementation may improve the memory in older adults.[61]

BLUING (HR)

A study respondent reported that bluing could be used to treat thrush. Bluing is a household product (containing a blue dye) that is used during laundering to improve the appearance of white fabric. Some white fabrics become yellowish after several washes, and adding blue dye causes the fabric to look white. No published information was found that supports the medical use of bluing.

BLUE STONE (HR)
(COPPER SULFATE, BLUE VITROL, BLUE COPPER)

Copper sulfate and other salts of copper have astringent action on mucus membranes, and in strong solutions it is highly corrosive. It is used as an herbicide, fungicide, and pesticide. It has been used as an emetic; however, it is too toxic to be used in this manner. Accidentally, consumption of copper sulfate has resulted in cases of severe acute toxicity.[62] **Copper sulfate should not be used for medical purposes.**

BORIC ACID (HR)

Study respondents reportedly used boric acid to treat tired eyes, pink eye, mouth ulcers, cold in the eye, and thrush. At one time, boric acid was widely used for minor eye problems.

It was sold in a 5% concentration with recommendations to dilute the purchased solution by 50% prior to use and discard the solution after use. The reason it was sold as a 5% solution is because bacteria will grow in it if the concentration is less than 5%. Although boric acid is not absorbed significantly from intact skin, it is absorbed from damaged skin, and fatal poisoning, particularly in infants, has occurred with topical application to burns, denuded areas, and granulated tissue. Serious poisoning has resulted from oral ingestion of as little as 5 grams.[63] Boric acid is used in the treatment of vulvovaginal candidiasis (VVC). The regimen is 600 mg of boric acid in a gelatin capsule inserted vaginally once daily for fourteen days. For resistant cases, it is used twice weekly for a longer duration.[64]

BREAD (BURNT) (HR)

Our study respondents reportedly used burnt bread (homemade activated charcoal) to treat vomiting. For years activated charcoal was used to treat accidental poisoning in children. In fact, a product containing one ounce of ipecac syrup and activated charcoal (universal antidote) was sold by pharmacies and kept in the home to use if accidental poisoning occurred. If activated charcoal was not available, burnt toast would be used instead. It was thought that the toast would absorb toxins from the stomach. No published clinical or scientific studies were found to support the use of burnt bread in this manner.

BROWN PAPER SACK (NEWSPAPER) (HR)

Study respondents reported that brown paper bags could be used to treat headaches, sties (eyelid sty), nosebleeds (newspaper), edema, and ringworms. Brown paper bags soaked in vinegar and placed across the forehead have been used to treat headache. Rolled newspaper was placed under the upper lip and held in place to stop nosebleeds. Wet ashes from burnt brown paper bags were used to treat ringworms. No published clinical or scientific studies were found to support the use of brown paper sacks for medical purposes.

BUCKTHORN (H)
(*RHAMNUS FRANGULA*)

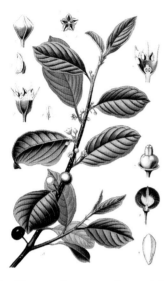

Study respondents reportedly used buckthorn for the treatment of fever blisters, constipation, penile discharge, foul smelling urine, rash, boils, bedsores, and warts. Buckthorn bark that has been aged for one or two years is used as a laxative. Buckthorn bark and berries are high in anthraquinone (stimulant) glycosides. Resins, tannins, and lipids make up the bulk of the bark's other ingredients. Anthraquinone glycosides have a cathartic action, causing the large intestine to increase its muscular contractions and increasing water movement from cells of the colon to feces, resulting in strong, soft bowel movements.[65] It takes six to ten hours for buckthorn to work when taken by mouth. When a laxative is needed a bulk form should be used. Dyes in buckthorn may turn the urine dark yellow or red. Buckthorn ointment has been used for warts and to stop itching. No published scientific or clinical studies to support the other listed uses for buckthorn were found.

BUTTER (HR)

Respondents reportedly used butter to treat burns and hemorrhoids. For many years butter was used to remove the tar after a person sustained a hot tar burn.[66] This treatment is no longer recommended. Cocoa butter, not butter, is a protectant commonly included in commercial products used to treat hemorrhoids. These products provide a physical barrier on the skin that helps prevent further irritation by liquids or stool. Butter should not be used to treat recent burns, and several effective nonprescription drugs are available to treat hemorrhoids. The currently recommended treatment for minor burns is to submerge the burned area in cold stagnant water until there is no pain in or out of the water.

BUTTERMILK (HR)

Respondents reportedly used buttermilk to treat cramps and ringworms. Buttermilk has been used to treat constipation and to replenish intestinal flora. Sour cream and buttermilk have been used to treat hives, ringworms, and other rashes. No published clinical or scientific studies were found to support the use of buttermilk in this manner.

CALAMUS (H)
(SWEET FLAG; *ACORUS CALAMUS* AND OTHER SPECIES)

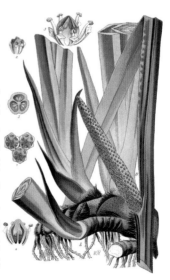

Study respondents used calamus to treat bad breath, toothache, chest pain, heartburn, nausea, cramps, gas, and worms. In the past calamus has been used to treat a wide variety of conditions. Infusions of calamus roots have been used to treat dyspepsia and fever. It is used for its sedative and tranquilizing effect.[67] Chewing of the roots has been used to treat indigestion and to clear the voice.

Calamus has also been used as a spice when cooking. There are four different types of calamus, and type I is American calamus. About forty years ago, feeding studies using calamus oil produced malignant tumors in the duodenal region of rats. Since the studies were conducted, the use of calamus as a food or food additive has been banned by the FDA.[68] However, a more recent study found extract of type I calamus had no significant mutagenic activity.[69] The plant and its extracts continue to be used throughout the world, and a recent study indicated that the extract may be useful in the treatment of cardiovascular problems.[70]

Calf Slobber (HR)

Study respondents reported the use of calf slobber to treat ringworms. When calves are suckling, they produce copious amount of slobber. The first author has witnessed the use of calf slobber to treat ringworms of the face. No published clinical or scientific studies were found to support the use of calf slobber in this manner.

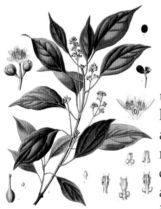

Camphor (H)
(Cinnamomum camphora)

Study respondents reportedly used camphor to treat headache, hearing loss (soften ear wax), toothache, cold sores, fever blisters, thrush, nasal congestion, cramps, menstrual cramps, acne, insect bites, muscle aches, arthritis, fever, bruises, sneezing, asthma, too much milk (while nursing), and vomiting. Topical camphor has been used as a counterirritant, antipruritic, and analgesic. It is also used to treat hemorrhoids, cold sores, warts, and arthritis. Camphor is frequently used for respiratory problems including inflammation of mucous membranes like nasal congestion and to suppress cough. It is also used for earaches and to treat minor burns. Camphor can be toxic when used orally and should only be used topically. The FDA and the American Academy of Pediatrics recommend that topical nonprescription camphor products not contain more than 11% camphor.[71] The American Academy of Pediatrics also recommends that camphor not be used in children. Additionally, topical camphor products should not be used on broken skin. Recently, acute toxicity of a ten-year-old who consumed three 100 mg nonprescription camphor transdermal patches was discussed.[72] One gram can be lethal to a child, and 20 grams can be lethal to an adult. Camphor is the active ingredient in several nonprescription drugs that have been approved by the FDA. However, published scientific studies supporting the use of camphor for many of the ailments listed above are lacking.

CARDAMOM SEEDS (H)
(*ELETTARIA CARDAMOMUM*)

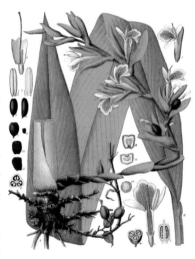

Study respondents reportedly used cardamom seeds to treat bad breath. They are also used to make cardamom products. They have a strong aromatic odor and an aromatic slightly bitter taste and contain no less that 4% cardamom oil. In traditional medicine, cardamom seeds have been used for a variety of ailments including acute respiratory disorders, stomach problems, hemorrhoids, bad breath, sore throat, colds, fever, bronchitis, gall bladder problems, flatulence, and colic. There is little or no published scientific evidence to support these claims. The seeds are primarily used in cooking.[73]

CASTOR OIL (HR)
(*RICINUS COMMUNIS*)

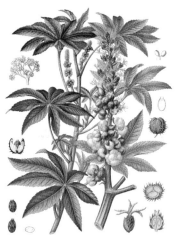

Study respondents reportedly used castor oil to treat pneumonia, vomiting, hernia, arthritis, and frostbite. Castor oil is the expressed oil from the seeds of the castor plant. It is used orally as a laxative, to stimulate labor, and to increase breast milk production. It is used topically and orally to treat arthritis.[74] It is also used topically to treat warts, to soften corns and bunions, to treat carbuncles, boils, abscesses, and other inflammatory disorders. It has also been used to treat migraine headaches and middle ear infections. Its use seems to be safe when used orally to induce labor at term,[75] but recent research investigating its effectiveness for this purpose was not supportive.[76] As a laxative, castor oil acts on the small intestine and can cause a fairly severe bowel movement. It also has a horrible taste that cannot be disguised by orange juice or coffee with cream and sugar. In most instances, if a bowel movement is needed, a bulk-forming laxative should be used. Published scientific studies supporting the use of castor oil for many of the listed ailments are lacking.

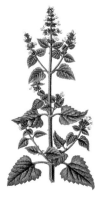

CATNIP (H)
(*NEPETA CATARIA*)

Catnip was used to treat thrush, bad breath, vomiting, and nervousness. Catnip traditionally has been used to induce urination and to expel worms from the body. It has been used as a sedative, to treat migraine headaches, nervous disorders, digestive problems, colds, flu, and fever. It has also been consumed as a tea to treat hives, and the stalk and leaves have been smoked to treat respiratory problems and to "get high." The validity of the reports regarding the euphoria properties are treated with skepticism by Tyler, et al.[77] Published scientific studies supporting the use of catnip for many of the listed uses are lacking.

CEDARWOOD OIL/TREE (H)
(CEDRUS ATLANTICA)

Respondents reportedly used cedarwood oil to treat asthma and dropsy. Cedarwood oil is a liquid distilled from the wood of cedarwood trees. The oil is frequently used to treat respiratory, skin, and urinary disorders. Cold and flu symptoms are sometimes treated with cedarwood oil. When vapor therapy with cedarwood oil is used, care must be taken to prevent damage to the mucous membranes. In a double-blind study, aromatherapy with cedarwood oil had no beneficial effect in the treatment of anxiety.[78] Published scientific studies supporting the use of cedarwood oil for many of the listed uses are lacking.

CELERY LEAF TEA (H)
(APIUM GRAVEOLENS)

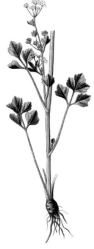

Respondents reported that they used celery leaf tea to treat dropsy, high blood pressure, constipation, gas, kidney problems, and arthritis. The beneficial health attributes of celery are ascribed to its seeds and oil. The oil and seeds are used orally to treat arthritis, hysteria, nervousness, headache, weight loss, loss of appetite, and exhaustion. Celery is also used as a sedative, mild diuretic, urinary antiseptic, digestive aid, menstrual stimulant, antiflatulent, and to reduce lactation.[79] There is little published scientific evidence to support many of these claims. Phytophotodermatitis has occurred in workers who cultivate or process celery.[80]

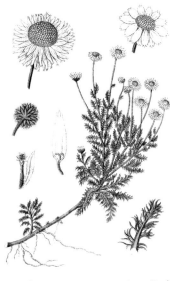

CHAMOMILE (H)
(ANTHEMIS NOBILIS)

Respondents reported that they used chamomile to treat heartburn and gas. Traditionally, chamomile has been used to treat digestive and rheumatic disorders. It has been used to treat worm infestations and to clean wounds and ulcers. Chamomile oil has been used to flavor cigarette tobacco, and it has been claimed to have anti-inflammatory, antibacterial, and astringent properties. It has been used to treat vomiting, colic, fever, and flatulence.[81] A recent study suggests that chamomile tea may have beneficial effects in the prevention of diabetic complications,[82] but topical application of chamomile has led to allergies in patients allergic to other plants in the daisy family, i.e., Asteraceae, or Compositae.[83] Published scientific studies supporting the use of chamomile for many of the listed ailments are lacking.

CHINABERRY ROOT TEA (H)
(MELIA AZEDARACH)

Chinaberry root tea was used to treat baldness and hair loss. Traditionally chinaberry bark has been used to treat roundworm, hookworm, and pinworm infestations. It has also been used to treat ringworm and other parasitic skin diseases. The authors found no published scientific evidence to support these claims.

Coconut Milk (HR)

Study respondents reportedly used coconut milk to treat cataracts. The respondents were using the liquid obtained from dried coconuts and incorrectly referring to it as "coconut milk." Traditionally, coconut milk has been used to treat colds, flu, sore throat, and a range of other illnesses related to the immune system. Coconut milk is claimed to be beneficial in the treatment of heart disease and atherosclerosis. The authors found no published scientific evidence to support these claims. An outbreak of cholera in Maryland in the early 1990s was traced to a contaminated imported shipment of frozen coconut milk.[84]

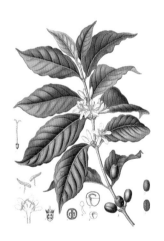

Coffee (H)
(*Coffea Arabica* and other species)

Study respondents reportedly used coffee to treat glaucoma, cataracts, and arthritis. Traditionally, coffee has been used to treat cataracts, and a recent study in rats indicate it may have some beneficial effects when used for this purpose.[85] However, the jury is still out. Coffee consumption was thought to increase the risk of developing rheumatoid arthritis, however, recent research did not support this finding.[86]

COHOSH, BLACK (H)
(CIMICIFUGA RACEMOSA, BLACK SNAKEROOT, BUGBANE)

Study respondents reportedly used cohosh to treat menstrual cramps and menopause. Black cohosh is used orally for the symptoms of menopause, to induce labor, for dysmenorrhea, dyspepsia, rheumatism, fever, sore throat, cough, as insect repellant, and as a sedative. Black cohosh is widely used and recently has been extensively studied.[87] Some black cohosh products appear to be effective in treating vasomotor symptoms like hot flashes associated with menopause.[88] Some case reports indicate that consumption of black cohosh may cause liver damage;[89] other reports do not support this finding.[90] Warnings have been issued against black cohosh use by women with a history of breast cancer, however, more recent literature reviews indicate the jury is still out on this issue.[91]

COHOSH, BLUE (H)
(CAULOPHYLLUM THALICTROIDES, SQUAWROOT, PAPOOSE ROOT)

Orally, blue cohosh has been widely used to induce labor, increase menstrual flow, and to treat other uterine conditions. It has also been used to treat rheumatism, epilepsy, and cramps. Several conflicting reports indicate that blue cohosh is teratogenic and is able to induce cardiovascular malfunctions in newborn babies.[92] According to a survey of midwives in the United States, approximately 64% reported using blue cohosh as a labor inducing aid.[93] Three case reports indicate that the use of blue cohosh at the time of delivery may have lead to prenatal stroke, acute myocardial infraction, profound congestive heart failure and shock, and severe multi-organ hypoxic injury.[94] The safety of the use of blue cohosh during lactation is also unknown.

COLA (HR)

Study respondents used cola to treat vomiting, heartburn, and belching. Flat cola has been used to treat nausea, diarrhea, and sore throat. The authors found no published scientific or clinical studies to support these claims.

COLTSFOOT (H)
(*TUSSILAGO FARFARA*)

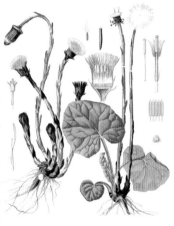

Study respondents reportedly used coltsfoot for the treatment of asthma. Traditionally, coltsfoot has been used orally to treat cough, sore throat, acute and chronic bronchitis, laryngitis, influenza, and lung congestion. As an inhalant, coltsfoot has been used for coughs and wheezing. Products containing pyrrolizidine alkaloids (PA's) like coltsfoot are unsafe when used orally. Repeated exposure to low concentrations of hepatotoxic PA's can cause severe veno-occlusive disease.[95] **Because of its toxicity, coltsfoot should not be used for medical purposes.**

COON FAT (HR)

Coon fat was used to treat hair loss. In the spring, summer, and fall, raccoons accumulate quite a bit of fat for use in the winter during periods of bad weather when they do not forage for food. It is this stored body fat that has been applied to the scalp to treat baldness. There is no published scientific evidence that this treatment is effective.

Corn Silk/Shuck Tea (H)
(*Zea May*)

Study respondents reportedly used corn silk/shuck tea to treat edema, menstrual cramps, back pain, and venereal disease (corn meal). A tea from corn silk/schucks has been used as a diuretic to treat all types of urinary problems, including inflamed prostate glands. It also has been used to treat diabetes and cardiovascular problems; however, published scientific studies supporting the use of corn silk/shuck tea for the listed uses are lacking.

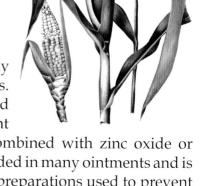

Corn Starch (H)
(*Zea May*)

Study respondents reportedly used corn starch to treat rashes. Corn starch is an absorbent and enjoys wide use as an ingredient in dusting powders alone or combined with zinc oxide or similar substances. It is also included in many ointments and is the primary ingredient in many preparations used to prevent diaper rash. Corn starch also helps provide protection against frictional injuries.[96]

Cream of Tartar (HR)
(Potassium Hydrogen Tartar)

Cream of tartar is a chemical derived from a crystalline acid deposited on the inside of wine barrels when the wine is fermenting. Cream of tartar and lemon have been used together to treat high blood pressure. It has also been combined with Epsom salt to treat arthritis, with water to treat urinary tract infections, and with sun-dried raisins to treat constipation.[97] Published scientific studies supporting the use of cream of tartar to treat high blood pressure are lacking.

CUCUMBER (H)
(*CUCUMIS SATIVUS*)

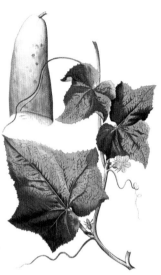

Respondents reportedly used cucumbers to treat edema, arthritis, and diabetes. Traditionally, cucumber has been used to treat high and low blood pressure, to cool and soothe irritating skin in patients with sunburn, and to provide fragrance in perfumes. The authors found no published scientific evidence that cucumbers are effective when used for medical purposes.

DANDELION (H)
(*TARAXACUM OFFICINALE*, NATURE'S COFFEE)

Study respondents reportedly used dandelion to treat arthritis (root), diabetes, and when feeling poorly (greens). Dandelion greens have been used in salads and in wine making and have been cooked like spinach. Dandelion roots have been roasted like coffee and used in herbal remedies to treat diabetes, disorders of the liver, as a diuretic, as a laxative and tonic, and to treat the common cold. Dandelion juice has been used to treat corns. Dandelion has caused contact dermatitis in susceptible individuals.[98] One preliminary study found that dandelion extract may have beneficial effects against prostate and breast cancer cells,[99] and a recent study reported that it lowered blood sugar.[100] Published scientific studies supporting the use of dandelion for the other ailments listed are lacking.

DEVIL'S DUST (H)
(TOAD STOOL)

Study respondents reportedly used Devil's dust to treat burns. Devil's dust is the spores produced by puffball mushrooms (Basidiomycota, gasterothecia) (gasteroid basidiocarps). The basidiocarps remain closed and open only after the spores have been released. They are called puffballs because a cloud of brown dust-like spores is released when the mature body bursts. Respiratory illnesses have been associated with the inhalation of puffball mushroom spores.[101] The authors found no published scientific evidence that Devil's dust is effective when used for medical purposes.

DOGWOOD (H)
(CORNUS SERICEA)

Dogwood was used to treat venereal disease. A tea made from its inner bark has astringent properties. The bark, flowers, and fruit are the parts of the dogwood tree that are used for their medicinal value. A drink from parts of the tree has been used to reduce fever, relieve chills, and as a remedy for colic. Extract of dogwood has also been used as an emetic. The authors found no published scientific or clinical evidence that dogwood is effective when used for medical purposes. Some members of the dogwood family may be toxic if consumed in large enough quantity.[102]

DUCKWEED (H)
(*LEMNA MINOR*)

Respondents used duckweed to treat vomiting. Reportedly, the whole plant has demulcent properties. It has been used in poultices. There is not enough published information available to determine if and how duckweed works for medical purposes.

EARWAX (HR)

Study respondents reportedly used earwax to treat sties, cold sores, and fever blisters. Earwax has been shown to reduce the viability of some bacteria and fungi.[103] Some of the bacteria are staphylococcal species that cause sties. However, no other published clinical or scientific studies are available that support the use of earwax for medical purposes.

EGG (YOLK/WHITE/SKIN/SHELL) (HR)

Respondents reportedly used the parts of egg to treat hair loss, pink eye, sore throat (whole egg), shortness of breath, ulcers (whole egg), abscess (skin), acne (skin), boils (skin and white), arthritis (white), and venereal disease (shell and white). Beaten whole eggs have been used to prepare a facial mask to improve the skin and as a shampoo to improve the appearance of the hair. Mixtures of egg white have been used to treat diarrhea in children, coughs, and hoarseness. Egg whites sometimes mixed with toothpaste has been used to treat minor burns. The skin of raw and boiled eggs have been used to treat boils, minor cuts, and bruises. Crumbled eggshell mixtures have been used internally to cut up worms in humans and animals. Eggs have been used externally for their cosmetic effect. Beaten egg whites have been used as a facial mask to make the skin look and feel smooth. It is postulated that the mask works because egg proteins constrict as they dry, pulling some of the dried skin cells with them, and when washed off some of the dried cells are also washed off. Although egg probably is effective for some of the uses described above, the authors found no published clinical or scientific studies to support the use of egg for these purposes.

EPSOM SALT (HR)
(MAGNESIUM SULFATE)

Respondents reportedly used epsom salt to treat headache, dizziness, tired eyes, pink eye, cold in the eye, dropsy, high blood pressure, edema, gas, corns, athlete's foot, abscesses, rashes, bruises, and infections. Oral magnesium sulfate is commonly used as a saline laxative and has been used for this purpose for many years. A more recent study indicates that nebulized magnesium sulfate can be used to treat acute asthma.[104] It also has been administered via the intravenous route to treat severe asthma attacks, but it should only be used as a second line therapy when used in this manner.[105] It is available as a topical application for the treatment of aches and pains. Topically, magnesium sulfate solutions have been used as a drawing (dehydrating) agent in the treatment of boils, carbuncles, and abscesses. It also has been used topically to treat acne and to remove blackheads. Hypermagnesaemia is uncommon after oral administration of magnesium salts except in the presence of renal impairment.[106] Published scientific studies supporting the use of epsom salt for many of the ailments listed are lacking.

EUCALYPTUS OIL (H)
(EUCALYPTUS—SEVERAL SPECIES)

Study respondents reportedly used eucalyptus oil to treat asthma. Eucalyptus oil has been used to treat the symptoms of the common cold and flu and is sometimes included in products like inhalants, lozenges, and liniments. It has an antibacterial inhibitory effect on pathogenic bacteria of the respiratory tract.[107] Inhaled eucalyptus oil vapor is used in the treatment of asthma and bronchitis. Topically applied eucalyptus oil liniment has anti inflammatory and analgesic properties.[108] Reports of toxicity after inhalation and/or topical application are not common, however,

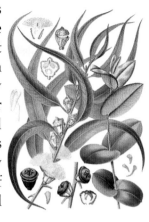

Deisinger, et al., reports a possible case of toxicity in a two-year-old attributed to the topical application of a eucalyptus oil liniment after a recent bath.[109] The amount of the oil needed to exert a toxic effect is unknown, but there are several reports of childhood deaths due to ingestion of pure eucalyptus oil, and eucalyptus oil should not be used in children.[110]

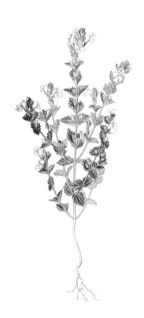

EYEBRIGHT (H)
(*EUPHRASIA OFFICINALIS*, EYE GRASS)

Study respondents reportedly used eyebright to treat tired eyes. Topically, eyebright is used as an ophthalmic eyewash for a variety of conditions, including conjunctivitis, blepharitis, eye fatigue, inflammation of blood vessels, eyelid and conjunctiva, and for inflamed eyes.[111] The safety, efficacy, and purity of eyebright have not been evaluated by the FDA, and its use in the eyes may be unsanitary and lead to eye complications. Therefore its use in the eyes is not recommended.

FAT MEAT/GREASE (HR)

Respondents reportedly used fat meat/grease to treat cold sores, pneumonia, boils, arthritis (grease), fever (grease), and frostbite (grease). The fat meat used for medicinal purposes by African Americans was primarily salt pork that had been preserved with large amounts of salt (sodium chloride). The grease that was used was grease excreted when salt pork with fat is fried at high temperature. Fat meat (salt pork) has been used to treat boils, to remove splinters, in place of tetanus shots after puncture wounds, and to treat nosebleeds. It is the salt in the meat that causes fluids to exit the wound, possibly carrying with it the splinter and/or Clostridium tetanus bacteria. Published scientific evidence supporting the effectiveness of fat meat when used for medical purposes is lacking.

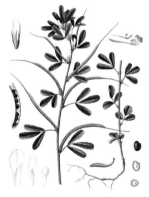

FENUGREEK (H)
(*TRIGONELLA FOENUM-GRAECUM*, ORIENTAL FENUGREEK)

Study respondents reported that fenugreek can be used to treat infections. The leaves of fenugreek have been used as an herb, and the seeds have been used as a spice and to increase breast milk production.[112] It has also been used for lowering blood sugar, weight loss, dyspepsia, gastritis, constipation, and high serum cholesterol and triglycerides. Several small studies show that fenugreek has some minor effectiveness in treating noninsulin dependent diabetes.[113] One study indicates that fenugreek seed extract has some effectiveness in reducing spontaneous fat intake in overweight subjects.[114] It has also been used orally for fever, mouth ulcers, boils, bronchitis, tuberculosis, chronic cough, baldness, and cancer. Topically, fenugreek is used as a poultice for local inflammation, gout, wounds, leg ulcers, and eczema. Published scientific evidence supporting the effectiveness of fenugreek when used for the other ailments listed is lacking.

FIG (H)
(*FICUS CARICA*)

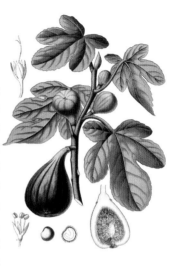

Study respondents reported that fig juice could be used to treat sore throat. Fig juice has been used for its soothing effect on irritated bronchial passages. This demulcent action is soothing to the inflamed mucous membranes that produce catarrh during a cold. Orally, fresh or dried fig fruit is used as a laxative, and it may be the small seeds in the fruit that causes an increase in intestinal contraction and bowel movements. Fig leaves have also been used to treat diabetes, hyperlipidemia, eczema, psoriasis, and vitiligo.[115] Other than the use as a laxative and for diabetes, the others medical uses are not supported by published medical evidence.

FLAXSEED (H)
(*LINUM USITATISSIMUM*, LINSEED)

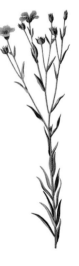

Study respondents reportedly used flaxseed tea for tired eyes, ulcers, and abscesses. Flaxseed is one of the best natural sources of alpha-linolenic acid. Flaxseed has been used to treat cough, colds, constipation, and urinary infections. Flax-seed oil is also used for dry eyes, as a laxative, and for rheumatoid and osteoarthritis. It is currently being studied for constipation, attention deficit hyperactivity disorder, breast cancer, menopausal symptoms, high blood pressure, HIV/AIDS, prostate cancer, and for its effect on blood lipids.[116] Published scientific evidence supporting the effectiveness of flaxseeds when used for the other ailments listed is lacking.

FLOUR (HR)

Respondents reported that flour can be used to treat nasal congestion, nausea, cramps, diarrhea, hemorrhoids, venereal diseases, and alcoholism. The authors found no published scientific or clinical evidence that flour is effective when used for medical purposes. Studies regarding the anti-cancer effects of the consumption of wheat bran are mixed and additional research needs to be done.

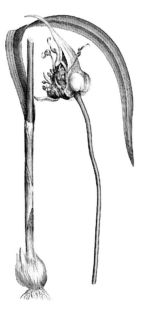

GARLIC (H)
(*ALLIUM SATIVUM*)

Respondents reportedly used garlic to treat blurred vision, high blood pressure, colds, gas, and worms. Traditionally, many medicinal values have been ascribed to garlic. It has been used to treat leprosy, deafness, earaches, flatulence, scurvy, atherosclerosis, high blood pressure, menstrual disorders, fever, coughs, headache, stomach ache, gout, whooping cough, hemorrhoids, asthma, bronchitis, worms, and shortness of breath. There is positive scientific evidence that garlic is effective for the treatment of high blood pressure, high cholesterol, and several other cardiovascular diseases. Evidence supporting its use for some of the other conditions listed is less positive.[117] There is insufficient clinical evidence to demonstrate that garlic is effective in the prevention or treatment of the common cold.[118]

GASOLINE (HR)

Study respondents reportedly used gasoline to treat arthritis. Gasoline traditionally has been used to treat chronic ulcers of the legs. Gasoline has also been used to treat head lice, and there are several reports of serious injuries from burns associated with the use of gasoline in this manner. It was also one of the ingredients in a topical capsaicin patch for the temporary treatment of minor muscle and joint pains. The FDA recently warned that there are no scientific studies to support the use of gasoline in this manner and that product was removed from the market. Additionally, there is no published scientific or clinical evidence that gasoline is effective when used for any medical purpose.

GINGER (H)
(*ZINGIBER OFFICINALE* ROSCOE)

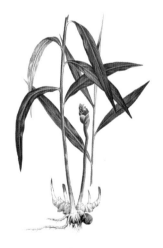

Ginger was used to treat cramps, menstrual cramps, irregular menstrual periods, muscle aches, and for abortions. Ginger has long been used as a spice. Traditionally ginger has been used to treat motion sickness, nausea, vomiting, flatulence, dyspepsia, loss of appetite, anorexia, colic, bronchitis, and for rheumatic complaints.[119] There is good evidence of effectiveness of ginger in the treatment of nausea and vomiting associated with pregnancy. Research also indicated that ginger is possibly effective in the treatment of motion sickness, postoperative nausea and vomiting, and vertigo.[120] Ginger has also been used to treat primary dysmenorrheal[121] and to treat knee pain associated with osteoarthritis.[122] Published scientific evidence supporting the effectiveness of ginger for abortions is lacking.

GINSENG TEA (H)
(*PANAX QUINQUEFOLIUS*)

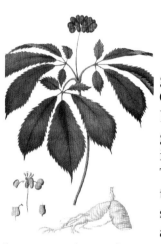

Study respondents reportedly use ginseng root to treat menstrual cramps. Ginseng has been used as a cure-all. Based on the "Doctrine of Signatures" ginseng's man-like appearance makes it useful for all of man's afflictions. Traditionally, ginseng has been used to increase resistance to environmental stress. It has been used to treat anemia, atherosclerosis, depression, diabetes, hypertension, edema, and ulcers. Research indicates that it is possibly effective in the treatment of diabetes[123] and respiratory tract infections.[124]

GLYCERIN (HR)

Respondents reportedly used glycerin to treat asthma. Orally, glycerin is a mild laxative and demulcent. It has been used for weight loss, enhancing exercise performance, and to reduce intraocular pressure. Glycerin is also included in many nonprescription medications including rectal suppositories.

GOAT'S MILK (HR)

Respondents reportedly used goat's milk to treat ulcers. Traditionally, goat's milk has been used to replace cow's milk because goat's milk casein and fat may sometimes be easier to digest than cow's milk. Recently, the FDA approved an anticoagulant (blood thinner) made from the milk of a genetically engineered goat.[125] Additionally, researchers are using goats to produce spider silk in their milk.[126]

GRAPE (H)
(*VITIS*—VARIOUS SPECIES)

Respondents reportedly used grape juice to treat diarrhea. Traditionally, grape leaf has been used to treat diarrhea, heavy menstrual bleeding, uterine hemorrhage, and canker sores. Pilot studies indicate that concord grape juice may be useful in treating nausea and vomiting associated with cancer chemotherapy; however, further studies are needed to confirm these preliminary results.[127] Additionally, another pilot study found grape juice effective in improving memory functions in older adults with mild memory loss.[128]

GUN SHELL POWDER (HR)
(POTASSIUM NITRATE, SALTPETER)

Respondents reportedly used gun shell powder to treat poison ivy. The gun shell powder the respondents used was a mixture of sulfur, charcoal, and potassium nitrate. Gun shell powder was used by slave traders to hide scars on slaves and increase their sales price.[129] One of the active ingredients in gun shell powder is potassium nitrate (saltpeter). It has been used topically to treat itching. It also has been used topically to treat small ulcers, wounds, and ringworms.[130] It has been used since the eighteenth century to treat asthma, sore throat, and arthritis. Along with sodium fluoride, it has also been used to decrease tooth decay in teeth sensitive to temperature, sweets, and acids or touch. It is one of the active ingredients in Sensodyne toothpaste used to clean sensitive teeth.

Hog Hoof Tea (HR)

Study respondents reportedly used hog hoof tea to treat pneumonia and influenza. Traditionally, hog hoof tea has been used for coughs and colds. Hog hoofs were boiled in water and the liquid consumed to treat coughs and colds. The authors found no published clinical or scientific evidence to support this use.

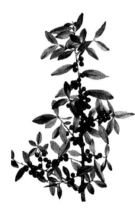

Holly (H)
(*Ilex*—Several species)

Study respondents reportedly used holly bush leaves to treat dropsy. Preparations of the leaves have been used as a diuretic, for cough, digestive disorders, fever, rheumatism, and as an antipyretic (to decrease body temperature). A tea made from holly berries has been used as a cardiac stimulant by American Indians. No scientific or clinical evidence to support the medical use of holly was found. **Eating holly berries can be fatal, especially for children.**[131]

Honey (HR)

Respondents reportedly used honey to treat hoarseness, asthma, bronchitis, pneumonia, tuberculosis, colds, influenza, and ulcers. Traditionally, honey has been used to treat asthma, to induce sleep, and cure diarrhea. Topically, it has been used for wound healing and to treat leg and foot ulcers. It is also used for the treatment of cataracts and postherpetic corneal opacities. Recent research indicates that honey is very effective when used to treat coughs.[132] If using on infants one-year-old or less, it should be refrigerated after opening because of the concern for botulism poisoning in this age group. Manuka honey, from New Zealand, has recently been found to have high antibacterial activity and is effective in the treatment of minor burns and other wounds.[133]

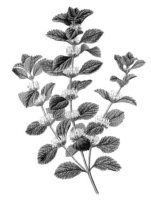

HOREHOUND (H)
(*MARRUBIUM VULGARE*)

Respondents reportedly used horehound to treat hoarseness and a cold. Traditionally, horehound has been used as a flavoring agent, expectorant, vasodilator, diaphoretic, diuretic, and for the treatment of intestinal parasites. Preparations containing horehound have been used to treat coughs and minor throat irritation.[134] It also has been used as a mild laxative. There is very little, if any, published reliable information available that supports the use of horehound for medical purposes.

HUCKLEBERRY (H)
(*VACCINIUM MYRTILLUS*, BILLBERRY)

Respondents reportedly used huckleberry root to treat venereal disease and the leaves to treat diabetes. In the past, huckleberry fruit has been used to treat diarrhea and scurvy. Currently, huckleberry is used orally for diabetes, menstrual

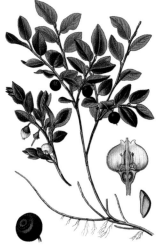

cramps, eye problems, varicose veins, venous insufficiency, and other circulatory problems.[135] There is very little, if any, reliable published information available that supports the use of huckleberry for medical purposes.

IODINE (HR)

Iodine was used to treat hair loss, hoarseness, goiters, and kidney problems. Iodine has traditionally been used orally to prevent goiters and as an expectorant. Topically, iodine is used as an effective antibacterial agent and skin disinfectant. It is also active against fungi, protozoa, cysts, and spores. It is used as an antiseptic and disinfectant generally as a 2.0% or 2.5% solution.[136] In its original form, iodine causes pain and irritation when applied to wounds, may impair the function of cells involved in healing, and discolors the skin. To decrease the pain caused by iodine when applied to wounds it has been combined with fats and proteins (odophors).[137]

IRON (HR)

Study respondents reportedly used iron to treat low blood pressure, edema, and bruises. Orally, iron has been used to treat iron deficiency and iron deficiency anemia, oral canker sores, depression, and to improve athletic performance. To obtain iron, home remedy users soaked nails in water and drank the resulting rusty solution. Very high doses of iron can be fatal in children and iron supplements must be kept out of their reach. The use of iron supplements in children should always be under the direction of a physician. Toxic ingestion of iron may be life threatening and should be referred immediately to a poison control center or emergency medical facility.[138] No published clinical or scientific studies were found to support the use of iron to treat low blood pressure, edema, or to improve athletic performance.

JIMSON WEED (H)
(*DATURA STRAMONIUM*, NIGHTSHADE, THORN APPLE)

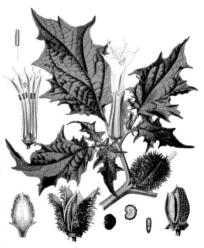

Study respondents reportedly used jimson weed to treat headache, asthma, pneumonia, rash, and poison ivy. Jimson weed has traditionally been used to treat asthma, cough, bronchitis, and influenza. Jimson weed contains the belladonna alkaloids, hyoscyamine, atropine, and scopolamine. Inhalation of the smoke from jimson weeds' leaves have been used to relieve spasms of the bronchioles during asthma attacks. Teenagers seeking a hallucinogenic high from the use of jimson weed have been hospitalized. Data from the American Association of Poison Control Center's national database indicates that annually an average of 427 individuals are poisoned from the use of jimson weed.[139] All parts of the plant, especially the seeds, can produce toxic reactions. **Jimson weed and its constituents should not be used for medical purposes.**

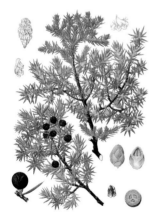

JUNIPER (H)
(*JUNIPERUS OXYCEDRUS*, *JUNIPERUS COMMUNIS*)

Juniper was used to treat colds. Traditionally, juniper has been used orally to treat worms, snakebites, kidney and bladder stones, loss of appetite, diabetes, acne, urinary tract infections, bloating, flatulence, dyspepsia, and heartburn. Topically, juniper has been used for rheumatic pain in joints and muscle, inflammatory diseases, and wounds.[140] Juniper is probably best known as the plant that gives the alcoholic beverage "gin" its distinctive flavor.[141] There is very little, if any, reliable published information available that supports the use of juniper for medical purposes.

KEROSENE (COAL OIL) (HR)

Study respondents reportedly used kerosene to treat toothache, colds, fever blisters, pneumonia, cold sore, hemorrhoids, cuts, arthritis, nervousness, and snakebite. Kerosene is primarily used as lighting fluid and heating oil and is mixed with other ingredients for use as a jet fuel. Kerosene has been applied to head lice, but this practice is painful, potentially dangerous, and should not be used. Kerosene and sugar has been used to treat colds, sore throat, cough, frostbite, diphtheria, and inflammation of the bowels.[142] Recently, a thirty-nine-year-old male who self-injected kerosene into his external hemorrhoids had a heart attack and died.[143] Ingestion of kerosene has lead to fatalities in infants and children. The prognosis of recovery is more bleak if aspiration (into the lungs) of the substance occurs. There is very little, if any, reliable published information available that supports the use of kerosene for medical purposes.

LARD (HR)

Lard was used to treat sties, dropsy, bronchitis, pneumonia, hemorrhoids, abscesses, scabies, arthritis, burns, snakebites, and frostbite. Lard is an emollient and has been used as a base in the preparation of ointments. Many years ago, lard was used orally to treat eczema,[144] and still is used in the preparation of lye soap. There is very little, if any, reliable published information available that supports the use of lard for medical purposes, excluding its use as a base in the preparation of ointments.

LEECHES (HR)
(*HIRUDO MEDICINALIS*)

Study respondents reportedly used leeches to treat black eyes. In 2004, the FDA approved the commercial marketing of medicinal leeches for medical purposes. The FDA approved leeches as medical devices, meaning they can be used in the diagnosis, cure, treatment, prevention, and mitigation of a disease or condition. Leeches have been used since the nineteenth century for a variety of ailments. The medical literature describes numerous cases of the use of leeches to relieve congestion following reattachment or transplantation surgery of fingers, toes, ears, penis, and other skin-flaps, in addition to breast reconstruction, reduction, or augmentation procedures where engorgement of the nipple can be complicated.[145] Currently, one of the primary uses of leeches is when an appendage with thin skin like a finger or toe is amputated and re-attached. When the appendage is re-attached, arteries that bring blood to the re-attached appendage develop approximately three days before veins do. If nothing is done, the re-attached appendage will drop off. If a leech is allowed to bite the appendage someplace beyond where it is re-attached, hirudin from the leeches' saliva will thin the blood throughout the body and a drop of blood will escape from the leech injury for about twelve hours. Leeches are used in this manner for about three days until veins develop. Hirudin is one of the most effective anticoagulants known to man. One of the major drug manufactures, using genetic engineering, copied hirudin, and has the patented drug on the U.S. market.

LEMON (H)
(*CITRUS LIMONIA*)

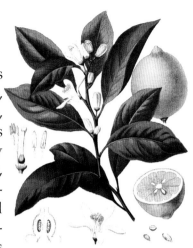

Lemon juice/lemonade was used to treat headache, hoarseness, high blood pressure, pneumonia, cold, nausea, vomiting, ulcers, loss of appetite, constipation, kidney problems, jaundice, arthritis, chills, fever, malaria, and diabetes. Lemon juice has traditionally been used as a diuretic, astringent, diaphoretic, tonic, and gargle.[146] Lemons have been used for scurvy,[147] the common cold, and to treat the flu. Topically, lemons have been used to treat acne, ringworms, warts, sunburn, and keloids.[148] There is very little, if any, reliable published information available that supports the use of lemon for most medical purposes.

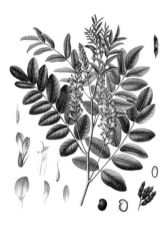

LICORICE (H)
(*GLYCYRRHIZA*)

Study respondents reportedly used licorice to treat menstrual cramps and menopause. Licorice is widely used in candy and as a flavoring agent. Licorice traditionally has been used to treat gastric and duodenal ulcers, cough, constipation, colic, dyspepsia, sore throat, bronchitis, tuberculosis, and contact dermatitis.[149] Two recent studies discuss adverse effects (black tarry stools in a warfarin patient and cardiac arrest in the other patient) of licorice when consumed by elderly patients.[150] Additionally, prolonged use of large doses may cause water retention, low potassium, and high blood pressure.[151] However, licorice candy sold in the U.S. is sweetened with anise oil rather than licorice and therefore does not cause these adverse effects.

LIFE EVERLASTING—SEE RABBIT TOBACCO

LIME WATER (HR)
(CALCIUM HYDROXIDE WATER)

Respondents reportedly used lime water to treat pinworms. Lime water has traditionally been used as an antacid, astringent, and antiseptic. It has been used orally for gastric irritation accompanied by nausea and vomiting. Externally, it has been used to clean skin ulcers. Lime water should be effective when used as an antacid and astringent.

LIVER (RAW) (HR)

Respondents reportedly used raw liver to treat black eyes. No published information discussing or supporting the use of raw liver for medical purposes was found.

LYE SOAP (HR)

Lye soap was used to treat poison ivy rashes. Lye soap is made from lye and lard and has been used to treat symptoms of psoriasis, eczema, and acne. It has also been used to treat rashes caused by poison ivy, sunburn, and bites caused by mosquitoes and chiggers. There is very little, if any, reliable published information available that supports the use of lye soap for medical purposes.

MANURE (COW) (HR)

Cow manure was used to treat fever. Stepping into a

fresh pod of cow manure has been used to treat athlete's foot problems, and dried cow manure has been boiled to make tea and used to treat colds and fever. Because lynching of African Americans males in segregated Mississippi was so prevalent prior to integration, many young African American males who lived there were taught at a very young age (four or five years of age) to use fresh cow manure in an attempt to evade tracking by blood hounds, when necessary. There is very little, if any, reliable published information available that supports the use of cow manure for medical purposes.

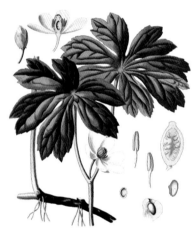

MAYAPPLE ROOT (H)
(*PODOPHYLLUM PELTATUM*)

Mayapple root was used to treat kidney problems. Podophyllum extracted from the roots of mayapples is a powerful laxative. The FDA had it removed from nonprescription laxatives marketed in the United States. Podophyllum has been used as a vermifuge to destroy and remove worms from the intestinal tract. It also is used topically as a prescription drug to treat anogenital and other warts. Podophyllum resin is very irritating to the eyes, skin, and mucous membranes and requires careful handling.[152] When used to treat warts, application to healthy tissue must be avoided. **Podophyllum should only be used under the directions of a physician.**

MERCUROCHROME (HR)

Mercurochrome was used to treat dental problems. Mercurochrome (Merbromin) is a topical antiseptic used for minor cuts and scrapes. Mercurochrome was not a very effective antiseptic, and in 1998 the FDA removed it from the "generally recognized as safe" and into the "untested" classification, thus stopping its distribution in the United States because of it mercury content. **Mercurochrome should not be used for medical purposes**.

MILK (HR)

Milk was used to treat tired eyes, ulcers, hernia, rashes, poison ivy, ringworms, and insomnia (used hot). Human breast milk has been used to treat pink eye, sore nipples, mosquito and ant bites, acne, eczema, diaper rash, stuffy nose, minor burns, and as a sexual lubricant. There is very little, if any, reliable published information available that supports the use of milk for any of these medical purposes

MILK OF MAGNESIA (HR)
(MAGNESIUM HYDROXIDE)

Milk of Magnesia was used to treat headache and vomiting. Milk of Magnesia is a laxative used to treat constipation and an antacid used to relieve indigestion, sour stomach, and heartburn. Topically, magnesium hydroxide is used as antiperspirant and to treat canker sores. It has also been used to treat acne, seborrhea, and dandruff. Milk of Magnesia is an effective laxative and antacid; however, published scientific or clinical studies supporting its use in the treatment of skin disorders are lacking.

MILKWEED (H)
(ASCLEPIAS—SEVERAL SPECIES)

Milkweeds were used to treat cuts and boils. A tea made from the roots of milkweeds has been used as a diuretic for kidney stones, as a laxative, and an expectorant. It also has been used to treat asthma, bronchitis, and to induce sweating. The sap of milkweeds has been used topically to treat warts, ringworms, and moles. Milkweeds contain cardiac glycosides, which if taken internally, can cause poisoning. There is very little, if any, reliable published information available that supports the use of milkweeds for medical purposes. **Milkweed is potentially toxic if large quantities are consumed.**[153]

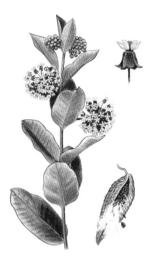

MOLASSES (HR)

Molasses was used to treat tired eyes, pink eye, earache, and cold-eye and colds. Molasses is the final solution found in the preparation of sugar by repeated evaporation, crystallization, and centrifugation of juices from sugarcane. Orally, molasses has been used as a vehicle for laxative medications like sulfur. Blackstrap molasses, the syrup obtained after the third boiling of sugarcane juice is a good source of iron, calcium, potassium, and magnesium. Molasses consumption may be useful in the prevention of anemia, osteoporosis, high blood pressure, and heart problems. It has been used to treat anemia associated with inflammatory bowel disease in an eleven-year-old male.[154]

MOTHBALLS (HR)
(NAPHTHALENE)

Mothballs were used to treat arthritis. An ointment made with lard as the base and mothball (naphthalene) as the active ingredient has been used to treat psoriasis and hair loss because of ringworms on the head. There have been several reports of adverse effects associated with the chewing and/or sniffing of mothballs.[155] There is very little, if any, reliable published information available that supports the use of mothballs for medical purposes.

MOUTHWASH (HR)

Study respondents reportedly used mouthwash to treat mouth ulcers, toothache, sore throat, and hoarseness. Traditionally, mouthwash has been used to treat cuts and burns, sore throat, poison ivy rashes, and fungal infections. There is limited scientific evidence that supports the effectiveness of mouthwash in the treatment of fungal infections or fighting plaque and promoting healthy gums when used on a short-term (two week to six month) basis.[156] It is of questionable value when used for the other ailments listed above.

MULLEIN (H)
(*VERBASCUM THAPSUS,* COMMON MULLEIN)

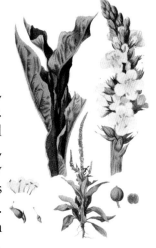

Mullein was used to treat edema, pneumonia, colds, chills, and fever. Traditionally, mullein has been used orally to treat hemorrhoids, gout, burns, and bruises. It has also been used orally to treat respiratory tract problems like asthma, cough, and tuberculosis. Topically, mullein leaves have been applied to soften and protect the skin. Yellow flowers from the plant have been used as a hair dye.[157] Recent research studies support some of the claimed beneficial health effects (e.g., tuberculosis) of common mullein.[158]

MUSTARD (H)
(BRASSICA ALBA, BRASSICA NIGRA)

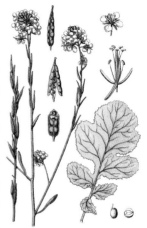

Respondents reportedly used mustard (leaves and dry mustard) to treat nasal congestion, constipation, and convulsions—epilepsy. Mustard is primarily used as a condiment, however its oil has been used topically to treat arthritis and as a foot bath for aching feet. Orally, mustard has been used as an appetite suppressant, emetic, and diuretic. The most common uses of mustard as a medicine are as plasters, poultices, and liniments. Mustard plasters have long been used to treat chest congestion from colds, influenza, bronchitis, bronchial pneumonia, sinusitis, pleurisy, lumbago, and sciatica. To make a mustard plaster, mustard seeds or powdered mustard with flour and warm water are mixed to make a paste. This mixture is spread between two pieces of cotton or linen and wrapped in flannel, then placed on the chest. Use of mustard plasters on the chest should be limited to ten minutes in adults and three minutes in children. Longer use may lead to blistering.[159] Mustard seed powder is currently being studied for it effect against bladder cancer.[160] Most of the evidence supporting the medical use of mustard is anecdotal.

NUTMEG (H)
(MYRISTICA FRAGRANS)

Nutmeg oil and powder were used to treat cramps and insomnia. The nutmeg tree is the source of the slightly different tasting spices mace and nutmeg. Mace is the dried part of the fruit of the plant and nutmeg is made from the seeds of the plant. Nutmeg is primarily used as a flavoring agent. Nutmeg and mace have been used orally to treat gastric disorders, including diarrhea, nausea, and flatulence.[161] Several reports of nutmeg intoxication have occurred when it was used for recreational purposes.[162]

OLIVE OIL (HR)
(SWEET OIL)

Olive oil was used to treat sore throat, pneumonia, hemorrhoids, kidney problems, dry skin, muscle ache, arthritis, hair loss, earache, fever blisters, and numbness. Orally, olive oil is best known for its cardiovascular health benefits, especially lowering cholesterol. Topically, olive oil was once marketed as a nonprescription product for the treatment of earache and softening earwax. A recently concluded randomized, placebo-controlled study found that olive oil had no beneficial effect on the perceived quality of sleep or the sleep-wake cycle.[163]

ONION (H)
(ALLIUM CEPA)

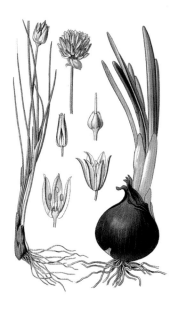

Onion was used to treat fever, colds, pneumonia, burns, corns, and calluses. Traditionally onion has been used orally to treat flatulence, whooping cough, fever, colds, cough, bronchitis, hypertension, angina, asthma, diabetes, and as a diuretic. Topically, onion has been used to treat insect bites, warts, bruises, furuncles, and to stimulate hair growth in cases of baldness. Results of a large epidemiological study indicate that daily consumption of onion may be inversely related to the development of pancreatic cancer.[164] Additional data suggests the higher the consumption of onions, the lower the risk for a number of types of cancers.[165] Consumption of red onion reduces blood glucose levels and may be helpful in the treatment of diabetes.[166] There is very little, if any, reliable published information available that supports the use of onion for the other medical purposes listed above.

PAREGORIC (H)
(CAMPHORATED TINCTURE OF OPIUM)

Paregoric was used to treat cramps. Traditionally, paregoric has been used to treat diarrhea in adults and children, as an expectorant and to treat cough, to calm restless children, and as a rub on the gums of children to counteract the pain of teething. The active ingredient in paregoric is powdered opium. Powdered opium is a very effective anti-diarrhea agent. Paregoric has also been used to treat the symptoms of narcotic withdrawal in neonates.[167]

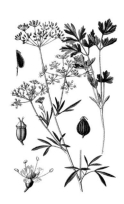

PARSLEY (H)
(PETROSELINUM SATIVUM AND PETROSELINUM CRISPUM)

Parsley tea was used to treat arthritis. Parsley seeds traditionally have been used to treat flatulence, colic, gallstones, and dysentery; the roots have been used as a diuretic and the juice to treat kidney ailments; the oil to regulate menstrual flow in the treatment of amenorrhea and dysmenorrhea; and the bruised leaves to treat insect bites, lice, and skin parasites. Other traditional uses reported are the treatment of prostate, liver, and spleen problems, the treatment of arthritis and anemia, and as an expectorant, laxative, and a scalp lotion to stimulate hair growth.[168] There is very little, if any, reliable published information available from human studies that supports the use of parsley for medical purposes.

PEACH (H)
(*PRUNUS PERSICA*)

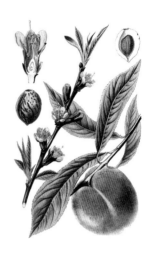

Peach (inner bark or leaves) was used to treat diarrhea (bark), chills (leaves), and fever (leaves). Traditionally, tea from the leaf taken orally and a poultice made from the leaves or bark is simultaneously laid on the stomach to treat vomiting. Peach seeds contain amygdalin, which breaks down to cyanide in the human body. Accidental ingestion of amygdalin is rare because the seeds must be crushed for its release. There is very little, if any, reliable published information available that supports the use of peach for medical purposes.

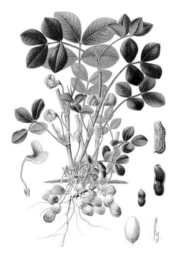

PEANUTS (H)
(*ARACHIS HYPOGAEA*)

Raw peanuts were used to treat diabetes. Non-honey coated or glazed peanuts are recommended as a low carbohydrate snack for diabetic patients,[169] and nuts, including peanuts, have been used orally to treat heart disease and to lower cholesterol. Topically, peanut oil has been used to treat arthritis, dry skin, and joint pain. Rectally, peanut oil has been used as an enema to treat constipation. Several cases of peanut oil allergies have been reported,[170] and in 2008, a peanut oil retention enema was discontinued in Europe.[171]

PENNYROYAL (H)
(*HEDEOMA PULEGIOIDES* AND *MENTHA PULEGIUM*)

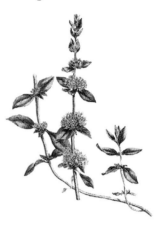

Pennyroyal was used to treat cramps and menstrual cramps. Traditionally, pennyroyal has been used orally to treat respiratory problems, as an abortifacient, to induce menstruation, and as an insect repellent and antiseptic. Pennyroyal should not be used during pregnancy. It should not be used to induce abortions because the dose at which it induces abortions is close to the lethal dose and deaths from its use in this manner have occurred.[172] **Because of its toxicity, pennyroyal oil should not be used for medical purposes.**

PEPPER, BLACK (H)
(*PIPER NIGRUM*)

Black and red pepper was used to treat sore throat (red), chest pain (oil), heartburn (black), diarrhea, menstrual cramps, abortion (black), and chills. Black pepper has traditionally been used to treat digestive problems, nausea, flatulence, diarrhea, constipation, and lack of appetite. It has also been used for the treatment of fever, rheumatic pain, hoarseness, insect bites, insomnia, and toothache. There is very little, if any, reliable published information from human studies that supports the use of black pepper for medical purposes.

PEPPER, RED (H)
(*CAPSICUM FRUTESCENS*, CAYENNE)

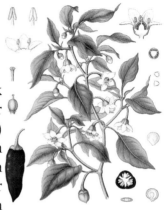

The reported uses of red and black pepper are listed in the Black Pepper entry above. Capsaicin (red pepper) ointments, lotions, creams, and skin patches available as nonprescription products have proven beneficial for many years in the treatment of pain due to arthritis, swollen or stiff joints, sprains, and backaches. Capsaicin has also been used to treat postherpetic neuralgic caused by shingles, as well as the symptomatic treatment of the pain from diabetic peripheral neuropathy.[173] Red pepper consumption has been shown to decrease appetite, decrease the symptoms of dyspepsia, decrease fat intake, and helps in the healing of gastric ulcers.[174]

PEPPERMINT (H)
(*MENTHA PIPERITA*)

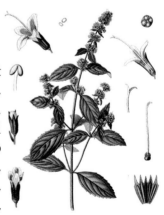

Peppermint was used to treat headache, dizziness, nasal congestion, hoarseness, chest pain, and nausea. Traditionally, oral peppermint and peppermint oil have been used to treat indigestion, nausea, vomiting, morning sickness, sore throat, colds, sinusitis, fever, cramps, dyspepsia, and flatulence. Topically peppermint oil, applied to the forehead and temples, is effective in the treatment of headache.[175] Recent research found that a peppermint gel was useful in the treatment of nipple cracking in breast-feeding women.[176] There is strong evidence of health benefits from peppermint oil for the treatment of irritable bowel syndrome.[177]

PERFUME (HR)

Perfume was used to treat toothache. Traditionally, essential oils (e.g., lemon, lime, vanilla, rose, and clove) have been used in making perfumes. Also, clove oil has long been used as one of the primary ingredients in preparations applied directly to a tooth or into a tooth cavity to alleviate toothache. Essential oils have a weak analgesic effect.

PETROLEUM JELLY (PETROLEUM) (HR)

Petroleum jelly was used to treat hair loss, cold sores, fever blisters, thrush, hoarseness, cuts, poison ivy, insect bites, acne, cuts, dry skin, ringworms, burns, vaginal discharge, and lack of vaginal lubrication. One of the primary uses of petroleum is as a vehicle for home remedies and pharmaceutical products. It is described in pharmaceutical textbooks as a hydrocarbon ointment base that is sometimes used without additional active ingredients because of its emollient properties.[178] It has been used to coat the teeth of contestants in beauty pageants to prevent lipstick from adhering to the teeth. It is useful to treat skin conditions where providing a mechanical barrier is needed (e.g., scrapes, cuts, burns, hemorrhoids, and anal fissures). Published clinical or scientific studies supporting the other uses listed above are lacking. Additionally, petroleum jelly should not be used as a vaginal lubricant because its mineral oil content will rapidly damage latex condoms.[179]

PINE (H)
(*PINUS STROBUS, PINUS MUGO, PINUS SYLVESTRIS*)

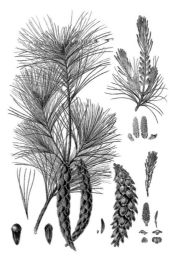

All parts of the pine tree have been used for medicinal purposes. Pine was used to treat bad breath, asthma, bronchitis, cold, tuberculosis, influenza, arthritis, bedwetting, and frostbite. Traditionally, pine has been widely used in inhalants to treat bronchitis and laryngitis. Pine needle tea has been used to treat coughs and colds. Pine needle baths have been used to treat cramped muscles and sore joints. Pine resin is used to make turpentine and externally the resin has been used to treat burns and sores. Pine tar ointment has been used to treat skin problems like psoriasis, scabies, and eczema. It has also been used to alleviate itching and peeling associated with sunburn. There is very little reliable published information available that supports the use of pine products for medical purposes.

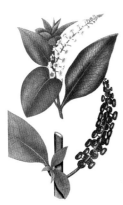

POKEWEED (H)
(*PHYTOLACCA AMERICANA*)

Pokeweed was used as a tonic. Traditionally, pokeweed has been used to treat many illnesses, including arthritis, tonsillitis, mumps, swollen glands, bronchitis, mastitis, constipation, fungal infections, joint inflammation, hemorrhoids, breast abscesses, ulcers, edema, skin cancer, and dysmenorrhea. **All parts of the pokeweed plant (leaves, roots, berries), are considered to be toxic, and the plant should not be used for medical purposes.**[180]

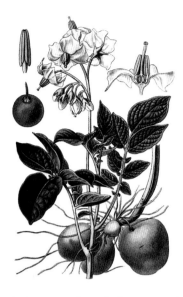

POTATO (H)
(*SOLANUM TUBEROSUM*)

Potatoes and potato peels were used to treat headache, black eyes, high blood pressure, and worms. Traditionally, raw potato poultices have been used to treat arthritis, infections, boils, burns, and sore eyes. Potato peel tea has been used to treat edema, and raw potato juice has been used to treat gastritis and other stomach disorders,[181] arthritis, gout, and eczema.[182] Green potatoes and potato sprouts contain toxic alkaloids and may cause severe poisoning if eaten.[183] There is very little reliable published information available that supports the use of potatoes for medical purposes.

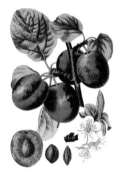

PRUNES (H)
(*PRUNUS DOMESTICA*)

Prunes were used to treat constipation. Dried prunes and prune juice have laxative properties and have traditionally been used to treat constipation. The consumption of a snack including dried prunes decreased feelings of hunger and desire to eat.[184]

QUININE (H)
(*CINCHONA OFFICINALIS*)

Quinine was used to treat headaches, hair loss, sties, abscesses, nervousness, venereal disease, numbness, chills, frostbite, miscarriages, and to induce abortions. Quinine has traditionally been used for years to treat malaria, fever, indigestion, cancer, and mouth and throat diseases. Quinine has also been used to treat leg cramps caused by vascular spasms. The FDA has issued a safety announcement indicating that quinine is only approved for use in the treatment of uncomplicated malaria and should not be used to treat night time leg cramps.[185]

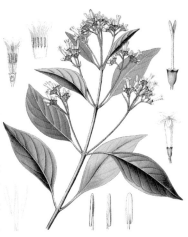

RABBIT TOBACCO (H)
(GNAPHALIUM OBTUSIFOLIUM, LIFE EVERLASTING)

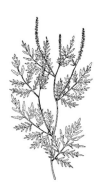

Rabbit tobacco was used to treat earaches, hay fever, and pneumonia. Traditionally, rabbit tobacco has been used to treat chronic coughs, bronchitis, diarrhea, flatulence, and colic. Externally, it has been used as a poultice to treat sprains, bruises, boils, and painful swelling. There is very little reliable published scientific or clinical information available that supports the use of rabbit tobacco for medical purposes.

RAGWEED (H)
(AMBROSIA ARTEMISIFOLIA)

Ragweed was used to treat chills. Preparations made from ragweed leaves have traditionally been used to treat diarrhea, intestinal disorders, ulcers, and hemorrhoids. The leaves were boiled in water and the resulting liquid was strained and used. For the treatment of diarrhea, intestinal disorders, and ulcers one ounce of the mixture was taken three times a day before meals. When treating hemorrhoids, a liquid prepared from the leaves is mixed with lard to make a salve. The salve is applied to the anal area twice daily.[186] There is very little reliable published clinical or scientific information available that supports the use of ragweed for medical purposes.

RASPBERRY (H)
(*RUBUS*—ALL SPECIES)

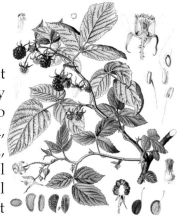

Raspberry was used to treat diarrhea. Traditionally, raspberry has been used to aid fertility, to increase the supply of breast milk, to control bleeding after childbirth, to regulate irregular menstrual cycles, to reduce heavy menstrual bleeding, to treat sore throat, to treat fever, and to treat canker sores. It was also used to treat diabetes, teething, colic, diarrhea, ulcer, prostate problems, gastric disorders, herpes, and gonorrhea. The use of raspberry leaf preparations during pregnancy have traditionally been recommended by some midwives. The efficacy of these preparations, when used in this manner, is not well documented, however, they appear to be safe under normal conditions of use.[187]

RED ALDER (H)
(*ALNUS RUBRA*)

Red alder was used to treat thrush. The bark has traditionally been used to treat headaches, coughs, stomach problems, asthma, eczema, poison oak, insect bites, and skin irritations. It also has been used to treat tuberculosis and lymphatic disorders. The stem bark contains two compounds (betulin and lepeol) that may suppress tumor activity.[188] There is very little reliable published clinical or scientific information available that supports the use of red alder for the ailments listed above.

RED CLOVER (H)
(*TRIFOLIUM PRATENSE*)

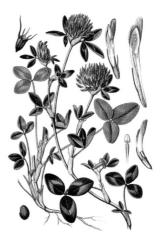

Red clover tea was used to treat back pain. Orally, red clover is used for menopausal symptoms and hot flashes, cyclic breast pain and tenderness, premenstrual syndrome, cancer prevention, indigestion, whooping cough, cough, asthma, bronchitis, and sexually transmitted diseases. Topically, red clover is used to treat cancer, skin sores, burns, sore eyes, eczema, and psoriasis. Although studies regarding the effectiveness of red clover in treating the vasomotor symptoms of menopause (hot flashes) are conflicting, a recent study found red clover to be effective in reducing depressive and anxiety symptoms among postmenopausal women.[189] Red clover contains phytoestrogens (plant estrogens) and therefore should be used only under the direction of a healthcare provider.

RED PRECIPITATE (HR)

Red precipitate was used to treat hair loss. Red precipitate is red mercuric oxide, and it has traditionally been used externally as an antiseptic to treat chronic skin diseases and fungal infections.[190] Newer and much safer medications are now used topically for fungal infections and chronic skin diseases. **Because of potential toxicities (mercury), red precipitate should not be used for medical purposes.**

Red Shank (H)
(*Persicaria maculosa*)

Red shank was used to treat venereal diseases. Traditionally, red shank has been used orally to treat diarrhea and infections. A preparation made from the leaves has been used to treat skin ulcers and sores and to stop bleeding. There is very little reliable published information available that supports the use of red shank for medical purposes.

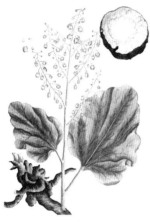

Rhubarb (H)
(*Rheum Palmatum, Rheum Rhaponticum,* and other species)

Rhubarb was used to treat heart-burn. The tannins in the root of the rhubarb plant give it laxative properties. In small doses it has been used orally to treat diarrhea and in large doses it is used to treat constipation. Topically, rhubarb has been used to treat cold sores and to stop bleeding.[191] Rhubarb is a very irritating laxative and there is very little reliable published information available that supports the oral use of rhubarb for any medical purposes.

Roman Cleanser (HR)

Roman Cleanser was used to treat corns, calluses, bunions, and athlete's foot problems. It is a sodium hypochlorite solution with actions described under the Bleach entry. **Roman Cleanser consumption is dangerous, and it should not be used for medical purposes.**

Sage (H)
(*Salvia Officinalis*)

Sage tea was used to treat diabetes, high blood pressure, anemia, hot flashes, menstrual cramps, hay fever, runny nose, colds, pneumonia, hair loss, and hernia. Traditionally, the tea has been used to treat digestive disorders, to control excessive sweating, dysmenorrhea, diarrhea, gastritis, flatulence, bloating, dyspepsia, and sore throat. It has also been used to treat depression, Alzheimer's disease, and for memory enhancement. It may have some effectiveness in the treatment of Alzheimer's disease.[192] Topically, it is used to treat minor oral injuries, gingivitis, laryngitis, and pharyngitis.[193] There are very few reliable published clinical or scientific studies available that support the use of sage for the other medical purposes listed above.

Salt (HR)
(Sodium Chloride)

Salt was used to treat tired eyes, pink eye, black eyes, cold in the eyes, toothache, fever blister, cold sores, thrush, mouth ulcers, hay fever, runny noses, nasal congestion, hoarseness, sore throat, sneezing, and nose bleed. Traditionally, salt solutions have been used for all of these purposes and topically to treat insect bites and stings, bee stings, and poison ivy/oak dermatitis. Short-term periodic use of normal saline solution is useful to treat nasal congestion. A recent study reported that daily use of normal saline solutions in the nostrils for a long period (twelve months) led to an increase in nasal infections.[194] Additionally, a salt solution is useful in the treatment of sore throat.

Saltpeter (HR)
(Potassium Nitrate)

Respondents reportedly used saltpeter to treat asthma. See the Gun Shell Powder entry.

Sardine Oil (HR)

Sardine oil was used to treat thrush. Sardine oil is one of the sources of fish oil that contains omega-3 essential fatty acids. It supports the cardiovascular system, functions of the brain, eyes, and the endocrine system. Fish oil also improves the health of the skin, reduces inflammation, treats rheumatoid arthritis, and lowers blood pressure. Sardine oil's effectiveness in the treatment of thrush has not been supported by published clinical or scientific trials.

Sarsaparilla (H)
(True Sarsaparilla—Smilax Aristolochiaefolia; American Sarsaparilla—Aralia Nudicaulis)

Sarsaparilla was used to treat venereal disease. Sarsaparilla has traditionally been used to treat skin disorders, arthritis, fever, colds, digestive disorders, leprosy, cancer, syphilis and other sexually transmitted diseases, minor burns, and insect bites and stings. From 1820 until 1910 it was listed in the U.S. Pharmacopoeia as a treatment for syphilis. There is little or no clinical research to support most of these claims. However, the anticancer value of the extract was more recently reviewed, and sarsaparilla may be effective against some cancer cells.[195]

Sassafras (H)
(Sassafras Albidum)

Respondents reportedly used sassafras oil to treat anemia

and colds. Traditionally the parts of sassafras used are the stem, leaves, flowers, pits, and roots. It has been used to treat pain, flatulence, to induce perspiration, as a diuretic, to treat gastrointestinal disorders, kidney disorders, liver disorders, eye disorders, colds, rheumatism, skin inflammation, insect bites, and lice. There is little or no published clinical

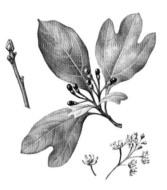

research to support most of these claims. Sassafras oil has been used as a flavoring agent for chewing gum, toothpaste, moonshine whiskey, and root beer. The main component of sassafras oil is safrole, which has been found to be carcinogenic when given to laboratory animals in large doses, and as little as 5 ml may be toxic in an adult.[196] The leaves of sassafras do not contain enough safrole to be toxic and are ground up (filé) and used to flavor gumbo.

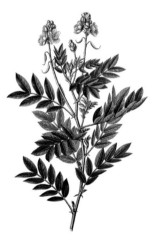

SENNA (H)
(*CASSIA MARILANDICA, CASSICA ACUTIFOLIA*)

Respondents reportedly used senna leaves to treat tiredness and constipation. Traditionally, senna has been used to treat constipation, hemorrhoids, and for weight loss. Senna is a potent laxative and is most appropriately used episodically. More recent reports regarding the chronic use of senna laxatives include heptotoxicity and perforation of the colon.[197] Extended use of senna should only occur under the direction of a healthcare provider.

Sloan Liniment (HR)

Sloan liniment was used to treat toothache. The active ingredient in Sloan liniment is capsaicin, which has analgesic properties. It is used topically to treat muscle and joint pain. It is also used to treat nerve pain in individuals who have shingles (see the Red Pepper entry). Capsaicin should be used topically in very dilute solution (0.75 to 1.5%) to prevent burning of the applied area. It should not be used on an area with thin skin and should be kept away from the eyes, mouth, and nostrils. It should also not be placed on dentures, contact lenses, and other items that come in contact with sensitive areas of the body.

Snuff (Smokeless Tobacco)—See Tobacco

Soot (HR)

Soot was used to treat cuts. Soot is a black substance formed by combustion or separated from fuel during combustion, rising in fine particles and adhering to the sides of chimneys or pipes conveying the smoke. No published information was found to support the use of soot for this purpose, and it should not be used.

Spearmint (H)
(Mentha Spicata, Mentha Veridis)

Spearmint was used to treat chest pain. Traditionally, it has been used orally to treat indigestion, flatulence, nausea, diarrhea, colds, sore throat, toothache, headache, cramps, and gallstones. It has been used topically to treat oral inflammation, arthritis, muscle pain, and skin disorders. Spearmint tea has also been used to treat hirsutism in females.[198]

It is useful in the treatment of minor gastrointestinal disorders like indigestion, but should not be used to treat chest pains, gallstones, and other more serious disorders.

SPIDER WEBS (HR)
(TELA ARANECE)

Spider webs were reportedly used by the respondents to stop bleeding. Spider webs have long been used for this purpose. The first author gives biweekly discussions and demonstrations on the "Use of Home Remedies and Herbals by African Americans" at one of the plantations in southeastern Louisiana. He frequently encounters elderly tourists from all over the world who are familiar with the use of spider webs to stop bleeding. In fact, he has used them on five occasions after suffering small puncture wounds, and they seem to work. However, the authors are not advocating the use of spider webs in this manner. Spider webs are similar to fibrin—a major blood clotting protein, but are somewhat less elastic.[199] Theoretically, spider webs may be potentially useful in stopping bleeding by replacing or enhancing the role of fibrin during blood clotting. There are no published clinical trials or scientific studies that support the use of spider webs in this manner. See the Goat's Milk entry for additional information regarding the use of spider webs.

STEAK (BEEF) (HR)

Beef steak was used to treat black eyes and to treat anemia. Traditionally, steaks have been used to treat black eyes, but should not be used for this purpose because of the potential of introducing bacteria in the eye area if the skin is broken. Anemia should be diagnosed by a physician prior to attempts to self treat it with medications, steak, or any kind of food, including black strap molasses.

SUGAR (ROCK CANDY) (HR)

Sugar was used to treat tired eyes, toothache, hoarseness (rock candy), asthma, colds, vomiting, heartburn, nervousness, worms, infection from leg ulcers, nausea, cramps, and bedsores. Rock candy is made by crystallizing sugar on a string or stick. Traditionally, sugar has been used orally as rock candy sometimes mixed with whiskey to treat hoarseness, cough, and colds. Also, sugar alone[200] or mixed with Milk of Magnesia, honey, and iodine has been used to treat bedsores. Sugar should be useful in the treatment of hoarseness, cough, and symptoms of colds. Published clinical and scientific studies to support the use of sugar for the other medical purposes are lacking.

SULFATE OF ZINC (HR)
(ZINC SULFATE)

Respondents reportedly used zinc sulfate to treat sties. Traditionally, zinc sulfate has been used for nasal congestion and for irritation of the eyes.[201] It also has been used topically as a deodorant. There are very few, if any, reliable published clinical or scientific studies available that support the use of sulfate of zinc for medical purposes.

SULFUR (HR)
(FLOWERS OF SULFUR, SUBLIMINAL SULFUR)

Sulfur was used to treat poison ivy, lice and scabies, hair loss, anemia, cold sores, and asthma. Traditionally, sulfur has been used orally as a laxative and to treat vomiting, diarrhea, headaches, insomnia, dizziness, and hot flashes. Topically, sulfur has been used to treat acne, dandruff, scabies, eczema, anal pruritis, hemorrhoids, and anal fissures. It also is combined with sulfaceamide and used in the treatment of rosacea, acne, and seborrheic dermatitis.[202] It is effective when used topically for skin disorders and when used internally as a laxative.

SUNFLOWER (H)
(*HELIANTHUS ANNUUS*)

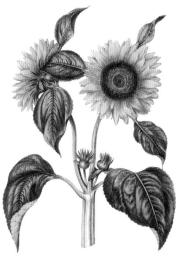

Sunflower was reportedly used to treat chills. Traditionally, seeds and the oil from sunflower seeds have been used to lower cholesterol and improve cardiovascular health. Sunflower seeds, oil, and leaves have been used for coughs and topically to prevent infection. Their solutions have also been used to treat bronchial, laryngeal, and pulmonary infections. Topically, sunflower oil has also been used to treat athlete's foot problems.[203] No published clinical or scientific studies are available that support the use of sunflower oil, leaves, or seeds for the treatment of chills.

SWEET OIL (OLIVE OIL)

See the entry on Olive Oil.

SWEET SPIRIT OF NITRE (HR)

Sweet Spirit of Nitre was used by the respondents to treat kidney problems and burning from urination. Although it was used to treat kidney and urinary problems for years, **its use was banned by the FDA in 1980, and it should not be used for medical purposes.**[204]

SYRUP (HR)

Syrup was used to treat earache (warm), sore throat, and burns. Traditionally, simple syrup has been used as a vehicle for medications. Syrups are concentrated solutions of sugar such as sucrose in water or other aqueous solutions. When purified water alone is used in making the sucrose solution, the solution is referred to as syrup or simple syrup.[205] Syrup should be soothing for the treatment of sore throat. Its effectiveness for the treatment of earwax and burns is questionable.

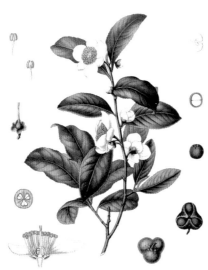

TEA (H)
(*CAMELLIA SINENSIS*)

Respondents reportedly used tea to treat tired eyes (tea bag), sty (tea bag), cold in the eye (tea bag), sore throat, asthma, for mothers with inadequate milk, cramps, menstrual cramps, and muscle aches. Traditionally, tea has been used to treat digestive disorders, insect bites, burns, gastrointestinal cancer, eye disorders, asthma, coronary artery disease, tooth decay, bad breath, diabetes, decreased urine flow, and headache. It is commonly believed that tea consumption has beneficial effects on cardiovascular health. Thus far, well-controlled studies have not been able to demonstrate these positive effects.[206]

THIAMINE (VITAMIN B1) (HR)

Thiamine was used to treat loss of appetite. Traditionally, thiamine has been used in the treatment of vitamin B1 deficiency syndromes, including beriberi. It has also been used to treat alcoholism, Alzheimer's disease, Crohn's disease, ulcerative colitis, congestive heart disease, depression, epilepsy, AIDS, canker sores, glaucoma, and cataracts. The use of vitamin B1 is effective in the prevention and treatment of problems associated with its deficiency. Published studies supporting the other uses of thiamine are lacking.

THOROUGHWORT (H) (*EUPATORIUM PERFOLIATUM*, BONESET)

Respondents reportedly used thoroughwort to treat tiredness. Traditionally, thoroughwort has been used to treat coughs, colds, fever, gout, arthritis, migraine headaches, worm infestations, malaria, influenza, and diarrhea. A tea made from the leaves and flowering top have been used as a laxative and emetic. **Thoroughwort contains ingredients that may be toxic and lead to liver damage.**[207] There is very little, if any, reliable published information available that supports the use of thoroughwort for medical purposes.

TOBACCO (H) (*NICOTIANA TABACUM*; CHEWING TOBACCO/SNUFF)

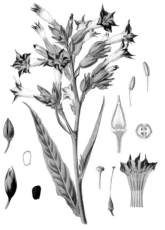

Tobacco and smokeless tobacco were used to treat earache (smoke) and insect bites. Tobacco has traditionally been used to treat pain, parasitic infestations, convulsions, colic, fever, insect bites, snake bites, toothaches, dizziness and fainting, to control sweating, and tuberculosis. It has also been used as a diuretic, as a poultice to treat boils and insect bites, vomiting, as a kidney aid for dropsy, and as a dermatological aid. An increased incidence of cancer of the mouth and gums, pharynx, and salivary glands in smokeless tobacco users has been reported.[208] It is questionable whether tobacco is effective for the listed ailments excluding insect bites, and it should not be used. A recent study found no detrimental effects of smoking on Crohn's disease and no clear beneficial effects on the course of ulcerative colitis.[209]

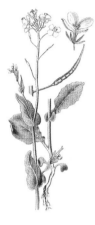

TURNIP (H)
(*BRASSICA RAPA*—WILD)

Respondents reportedly used wild turnips to treat sore throat, garden turnips to treat constipation, and roasted turnips to treat frostbite. Traditionally, turnips have been used to treat bronchial conditions like asthma, coughs, colds, and runny nose. There is very little reliable published information available that supports the use of turnips for medical purposes.

TURPENTINE (H)
(*TEREBINTHINA VULGARIS*, COMMON AMERICAN TURPENTINE)

Respondents reportedly used turpentine to treat cold sores, fever blisters, nasal congestion, sore throat, hoarseness, pneumonia, colds, corns, acne, insect stings, lice, boils, toothache, muscle aches, hemorrhoids, cramps, menstrual cramps, vaginal discharge, abortion, arthritis, worms, snake bites, and insect bites. It has traditionally been used orally to treat colds and as a diuretic, a stimulant, a laxative, and mixed with sugar to treat intestinal parasites. It has been used as an inhalant for nasal and throat ailments. Topically, it has been used to treat arthritis, burns, and sores. Recent reports regarding the adverse effects of turpentine use include occupational asthma,[210] allergic contact dermatitis,[211] lung necrosis in a toddler,[212] and acute intoxication and recovery after consumption of a massive dose.[213] There is very little reliable published information available that supports the use of turpentine for medical purposes.

URINE (MALE) (HR)

Male urine was used to treat earache and sore throat. Urine therapy has traditionally been used to treat arthritis, eczema, psoriasis, diabetes, multiple sclerosis, herpes, snakebites, and jellyfish and bee stings. Proponents of urine therapy indicate that for internal use the morning's first urine production should be used, and for external use new or old urine can be used. They indicate that since old urine has a higher concentration of ammonia, it is more effective against skin diseases and rashes. Although there is no published scientific research to support the use of urine in this manner, for years, ammonia has been a common ingredient in products used to treat skin diseases and rashes.

VANILLA (FLAVORING/EXTRACT) (H)

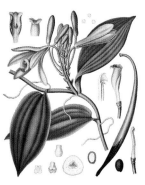

Respondents reportedly used vanilla flavoring to treat toothache. Traditionally, vanilla flavoring/extract has been used as an aphrodisiac, an antipyretic, as a stimulant, and to treat depression. It also has long been used to prevent dental caries, however vanilla can cause tooth surface loss.[214] Essential oils like clove oil have been used for years to treat toothache and were the active ingredients in many nonprescription products sold for this purpose. Vanilla may also be beneficial in the treatment of sickle cell anemia.[215]

Vicks VapoRub (HR)

Respondents reportedly used Vicks VapoRub to treat headache, cold sores, fever blisters, asthma, bronchitis, pneumonia, hemorrhoids, and vaginal discharge. Vicks VapoRub has been taken orally to treat coughs and colds. It also has been rubbed on the chest, nose, and throat for the same purpose. It has been applied to the sole of the feet to treat cough, applied to the toenails to treat fungal infections, and it has been used for jock itch. In a recent study, Vicks VapoRub was found to improve cold symptoms in children.[216] Reportedly, Vicks VapoRub can also cause too much mucus secretion and breathing problems when it is used in infants and babies.[217] Additionally, allergic contact dermatitis has been reported from exposure to its components.[218] Vicks VapoRub, applied topically, may be useful in the treatment of symptoms related to colds. Vick's VapoRub may be effective in the treatment of toenail fungus (onychomycosis). A study of eighteen individuals found that 83 percent showed benefit; over 25 percent were cured after forty-eight weeks of applying Vick's VapoRub to affected toenails and another 55 percent showed partial clearance. All eighteen individuals indicated they were satisfied or very satisfied with the appearance of their nails after treatment.[219] Published studies supporting the other uses listed above are lacking.

Vinegar (HR)

Respondents reportedly used vinegar to treat headaches, dizziness, sore throat, colds, hoarseness, blood pressure, chest pain, edema, heartburn, nausea, gas, corns, arthritis, sprains, menstrual cramps, vaginal discharge, and feminine cleansing. One treatment reported for headache was to soak strips of brown paper bags in vinegar, wrap the strips around the forehead, and let them dry and tighten to relieve the headache.

Vinegar is diluted acetic acid. It has traditionally been used to cool sunburns, to treat itching, burns, coughs, colds, hiccups, sore throat, bladder infections, infections, leg cramps, arthritis, sprained muscles, corns, calluses, sore feet, fungal infections of the nails, indigestion, heartburn, nausea, high blood pressure, high cholesterol, and memory loss. Diluted acetic acid has been used as an antibacterial, antifungal, and anti-protozoal in vaginal gels and douches, irrigations, topical preparations for skin and nails, and in ear drops. Diluted vinegar has also been used as an expectorant and as astringent lotion. Vinegar or 3-10% acetic acid solutions are sometimes applied to box jellyfish stings to inactivate any fragments of tentacles.[220] Vinegar may cause discharge of tentacles in some species of jellyfish (Man-of-War).[221]

VITAMIN E (VITAMIN E OIL) (HR)

Vitamin E was used to treat ingrown toenails, cuts, and impotence. Traditionally, vitamin E has been used orally to treat vitamin E deficiency, Alzheimer's disease, Parkinson's disease, night cramps, restless leg syndrome, anemia, angina, atherosclerosis, bladder cancer, breast cancer, and other types of cancer. Topically, vitamin E has been used to treat dark circles under the eyes, sunburn, cold sores, psoriasis, eczema, acne scars, and sexual arousal disorders. Orally, vitamin E is effective in the treatment of vitamin E deficiency, and it may be effective in the treatment of dementia and Alzheimer's disease.[222] Recent research found that men who took four hundred international units of vitamin E daily had more prostate cancer than men who took a placebo. Based on these results, men should not take oral vitamin E supplements for the prevention or treatment of prostrate cancer.[223] However, there is very little reliable published information available that supports the use of vitamin E for the other ailments listed above.

WALNUT (H)
(*JUGLANS REGIA*, ENGLISH WALNUT; *JUGLANS CINERA*, WHITE WALNUT, BUTTERNUT; *JUGLANS NIGRA*, BLACK WALNUT)

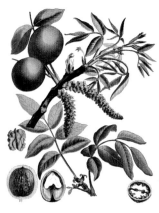

Reportedly, respondents used walnut to treat ringworm and jaundice. Bark of walnuts have traditionally been used to treat diarrhea, dysentery, soreness of the mouth, inflamed tonsils, and skin diseases, and to decrease milk production in weaning mothers. Walnut nuts have been used to stop vomiting during pregnancy, to calm hysteria, and to treat herpes. The ground hull of the nut has been used for head and body lice, herpes, internal parasites, liver flukes, and skin diseases. Walnut leaves have been used to treat boils, eczema, hives, skin ulcers, and sores. Diluted walnut oil has been used to treat colic, dandruff, and gangrene. The green rinds of the fruit have been used to treat ringworms. A recent meta-analysis of thirteen short-term studies indicated that high consumption of walnuts may decrease total and LDL cholesterol.[224] There is very little reliable published clinical information available that supports the use of walnut for most of the ailments listed.

WATERMELON (H)
(*CITRULLUS VULGARIS*)

Watermelon seeds were used to treat vaginal discharge and kidney problems and the rind to treat poison ivy. Traditionally, watermelon seed tea has been used to stimulate the functioning of the bladder and kidneys. It has also been used for the relief of flatulence and for ovarian inflammation due to accumulation of fluids in the lower abdominal region or pelvic region. Watermelon seed tea has been used to dissolve kidney stones and lower blood pressure. An earlier study that indicated that consumption of watermelon may enhance male erections was not supported by a follow-up study.[225] There is very little reliable published clinical information available that supports the use of watermelon for most of the ailments listed.

WHISKEY (HR)

Respondents reportedly used whiskey to treat headache, hair loss, thrush, sore throat, asthma, fever, pneumonia, colds, cramps, constipation, and anemia. Prior to the development of most analgesics, whiskey was used to relieve pain. It has also been used to prevent infections by fungi, bacteria, and many viruses. For additional uses of whiskey see the Alcohol entry.

WITCH HAZEL (H)
(*HAMAMELIS VIRGINIANA*)

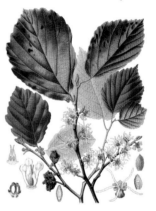

Respondents reportedly used witch hazel to treat tired eyes, black eyes, eye-cold, rashes, poison ivy, acne, tender breast, and feminine cleansing. Witch hazel tinctures have traditionally been used as a treatment for skin disorders and as a tonic for various medical conditions (e.g., diarrhea, vomiting blood, coughing up blood, tuberculosis, colds, fever, and cancer). The leaves, stems, and bark contain tannins; these agents may have astringent, hemostatic, venotonic, and anti-irritant/anti inflammatory properties. Topically, witch hazel is used to treat itching, skin inflammation, hemorrhoids, varicose veins, insect bites, and minor skin injuries and burns. Witch hazel is a component of many nonprescription hemorrhoid preparations. Used topically witch hazel may be somewhat effective; however, there is very little reliable published clinical information available that supports the use of witch hazel for most of the other conditions listed.[226]

GLOSSARY

(Definitions primarily from 1) Stedman's *Medical Dictionary*; 21st edition, 1966; Williams and Wilkins; Baltimore 2) Stedman's *Medical Dictionary for the Health Professions and Nursing*, 7th edition, 2011; Williams and Wilkins Philadelphia, Baltimore, New York, London, Buenos Aries, Hong Kong and Tokyo: and medical and pharmaceutical textbooks)

Anthraquinone: the basis of natural cathartic (laxative) principles in plants

Anticoagulant: an agent that prevents coagulation (blood clotting)

Antipruritic: an agent that prevents or relives itching

Antipyretic: an agent that reduces fever

Aspiration: removal, by suction, of air or fluid from a body cavity, from a region where unusual collections have accumulated

Atherosclerosis: deposits of lipid (fat) materials in arteries leading to major organs with subsequent reduction in blood flow to the organ

Astringent: an agent that causes contraction of tissues, arrest of secretion, or control of bleeding

Blepharitis: inflammation of the eyelids

Cathartic: an agent that causes active movement of the bowels

Catarrh: simple inflammation of a mucous membrane

Compendium: a summary or abstract containing the essential information in a brief form

Counterirritant: an agent that causes irritation or mild inflammation of the skin with the objective of relieving a deep-seated inflammatory process

Demulcent: an agent that soothes or relieves irritation especially of the mucous membrane

Diabetic peripheral neuropathy: damage to the peripheral nervous system caused by diabetes

Dropsy: an excessive accumulation of clear watery fluid in any of the tissues or cavities of the body

Dysmenorrhea: difficult and painful menstruation

Eczema: an inflammation of the skin of acute or chronic nature

Emollient: an agent that softens or soothes the skin or mucous membrane

Essential oil: a volatile oil from a plant

Expectorant: an agent that increases bronchial secretion and facilitates its expulsion

Fatty Acid: any acid that in combination with glycerin forms fat

Glycoside: the condensation product of a sugar with any other organic grouping by way of an ether link involving the reducing carbon of the sugar

Goiter: a chronic enlargement of the thyroid gland, not due to a neoplasm (tumor), frequently caused by a deficiency in dietary iodine

Hepatic veno-occlusive disease: a condition in which some of the small veins in the liver are blocked

Hirsutism: excessive facial hair growth

Hydrocarbon: a compound containing only hydrogen and carbon

Intraocular: within the eyeball

Iodophors: are combinations of iodine with carrier agents

Keloid: a scarring skin condition

Linolenic Acid: an unsaturated fatty acid, essential in nutrition

Lupus: a disease of the skin and mucous membrane

Manuka tree: a New Zealand tree in which honeybees build their hives

Meta-analysis: a method designed to increase the reliability of research by combining and analyzing the results of several studies of the same product or experiments on the same subject

Mucous membranes: membranes that line all internal

body cavities

Nebulize: to break up a liquid into a fine spray or vapor

Oleoresin: a compound of an essential oil and resin, present in certain plants

Podophyllum: the Mayapple or American Mandrake plant

Poultice: a hot, soft, moist mass, as of flour, herbs, mustard, etc., sometimes spread on cloth, applied to a sore or inflamed part of the body

Posthepatic neuralgic: a neuralgia (nerve pain) caused by the varicella zoster virus that typically follows an outbreak of herpes zoster (shingles)

Protectant: a substance applied to a surface in order to protect it from damage or injury

Purposive: serving some purpose

Pyrrolizidine Alkaloids: a group of naturally occurring alkaloids produced by certain plants that, when taken internally, cause liver damage (hepatic veno-occlusive disease)

Resin: an amorphous brittle substance consisting of the harden secretion of a number of plants, sometimes derived from a volatile oil

Rosacea: inflammation of the nose and cheeks associated with papules, pustules, and dilated blood vessels

Seborrheic Dermatitis: dermatitis caused by over activity of the sebaceous glands

Urticaria: an eruption of itching wheals usually of systemic origin

Tannin: tannic acid — an acid extracted from gall and used as an astringent

Unsaturated fatty acid: a fatty acid with a carbon chain that possesses one or more double or triple bond. They can absorb additional hydrogen

Warfarin: a prescription medication widely used to prevent blood clots

Wheal: an acute, circumscribed, swollen area of the skin

REFERENCES

1. Common Health Care beliefs and Practices of Puerto Ricans, Haitians, and Low Income Blacks in the New York/New Jersey Area. New York: The John Snow Public Health Group; 1983; Taylor SD, Boyd EL, Shimp LA. A review of home remedy use among African Americans. *Afr Am Res Prospect.* 1998; 48: 126-134.

2. Webster's New World College Dictionary. Indianapolis, IN: Wiley Publishing Company; 2002.

3. Harry Heller Research Corporation. Health Care Practices and Perceptions: A consumer Survey of Self-Medication. Washington, DC: The Proprietary Association; 1984; Harry Heller Research Corporation. Self-medication in the 90s: Practices and perceptions. Washington, DC: Nonprescription Drug Manufacturers Association; 1992.

4. Harry Heller Research Corporation. Health Care Practices and Perceptions.

5. Harry Heller Research Corporation. Self-medication in the 90s.

6. Barnes PM, Powell-Griner E, McFann K, Nahin RL. Complementary and alternative medicine use among adults: United States. 2004; 343: 1-19.

7. Ibid.

8. Barnes PM, Bloom B, Nahin RL. Complementary and alternative medicine use among adults and children: United States. 2007; 12: 1-23.

9. Boyd EL, Shimp LA, Hackney MJ. Home Remedies and the Black Elderly: a Reference Manual for Health Care Providers. Ann Arbor, MI: Institute of Gerontology and the College of Pharmacy; 1984; Boyd EL, Taylor SD, Shimp LA, Semler CR. An Assessment of home remedy use by African Americans. *J Natl Med Assoc.* 2000; 92: 341-353.

10.   Boyd EL, Shimp LA, Hackney MJ. Home Remedies and the Black Elderly.

11.   Current Population Survey. US Census Bureau, Department of Commerce. Washington, DC; 2003.

12.   Rollings-Magnusson S. Flaxseed, goose grease, and gun powder: medical practices by women homesteaders in Saskatchewan (1882-1914). *J Fam Hist*. 2008; 33: 388-410.

13.   Jackson JS, Gurin G. National Survey of Black Americans, Wave 1, 1979-1980 (computer file) Conducted by the University of Michigan Survey Research Center ICPSR ed. Ann Arbor, MI: Inter-University Consortium for Political and Social Research; 1996.

14.   Boyd EL, Taylor SD, Shimp LA, Semler CR. An Assessment of home remedy use by African Americans.

15.   Snow LF. Folk medical beliefs and their implications for care of patients: a review based on studies among Black Americans. Ann Inter Med. 1974; 81: 82-96; Stewart H. Kindling of hope in the disadvantaged; a study of Afro-American healers. *Mental Hyg*. 1971; 55: 96-100.

16.   Boyd EL, Taylor SD, Shimp LA, Semler CR. An Assessment of home remedy use by African Americans; Stewart H. Kindling of hope in the disadvantaged.

17.   Snow LF. Folk medical beliefs and their implications for care of patients; Stewart H. Kindling of hope in the disadvantaged; Murphree AH, Barrow MV. Physician dependence self-treatment practices, and folk remedies in a rural area. *South Med J*. 1970; 63: 403-408.

18.   Boyd EL, Shimp LA, Hackney MJ. Home Remedies and the Black Elderly; Snow LF. Folk medical beliefs and their implications for care of patients; Banahan BF, Frate DA. Use of home remedies and over-the-counter products among rural residents at risk for development of coronary heart disease. Paper presented at the (139th) American Pharmaceutical Association Annual Meeting. March 14-18, 1992. San Diego, CA; 1992; Appelt GD, Appelt JM. Perspectives of herb use in Hispanic folk medicine in the San Luis Valley of Colorado, USA. *Social Pharmacol*; 1987: 41-56.

19.   Boyd EL, Shimp LA, Hackney MJ. Home Remedies and the Black Elderly; Appelt GD, Appelt JM. Perspectives of herb use in Hispanic folk medicine.

20. Snow LF. Folk medical beliefs and their implications for care of patients; Stewart H. Kindling of hope in the disadvantaged.

21. Ibid.

22. Boyd EL, Shimp LA, Hackney MJ. Home Remedies and the Black Elderly; Appelt GD, Appelt JM. Perspectives of herb use in Hispanic folk medicine.

23. Common Health Care beliefs and Practices of Puerto Ricans, Haitians, and Low Income Blacks in the New York/New Jersey Area; Boyd EL, Shimp LA, Hackney MJ. Home Remedies and the Black Elderly; Snow LF. Folk medical beliefs and their implications for care of patients; Chesney AP, Thompson BL, Guevara A, Vela A, Scottstaedt MF. Mexican-American folk medicine implications for the family physician. *J Fam Pract.* 1980; 11: 567-574.

24. Eisenberg DM. Advising patients who seek alternative medical therapies. *Ann Intern Med.* 1997; 127: 61-69; Eisenberg DM, Kessler RC, Foster C, Norlock FE, Calkins DR, Delbanco TL. Unconventional medicine in the United States; prevalence, costs, and patterns of use. *N Engl J Med.* 1993; 328: 246-252.

25. Snow LF. Folk medical beliefs and their implications for care of patients.

26. Boyd EL, Shimp LA, Hackney MJ. Home Remedies and the Black Elderly; Murphree AH, Barrow MV. Physician dependence self-treatment practices.

27. Stewart H. Kindling of hope in the disadvantaged.

28. Banahan BF, Frate DA. Use of home remedies and over-the-counter products.

29. Osol A, Hoover, J E. Remington's Pharmaceutical Sciences, 15th ed. Easton, PA: Mack Publishing Co.; 1975. p. 1093.

30. Parfitt K. *Martindale: The Complete Drug Reference.* 32nd ed. London: The Pharmaceutical Press; 1999. p. 1118.

31. Hwang J, Hodis HN, Sevanien A. Soy and alfalfa phytoestrogen extracts becomes potent lipo-protein antioxidants in the presence acerola

cherry extract. *J Agric Food Chem.* 2001; 49: 308-314.

32. Molgaard J, von Schenck H, Olsen AG. Alfalfa seeds lower low density lipoprotein cholesterol and apolipoprotein B concentrations in patients with type II hyperlipoproteinemia. *Atherosclerosis.* 1987; 21:173-179.

33. Malinow MR, Bardana EJ Jr, Goodnight AJ Jr. Pancytopeina during ingestion of alfalfa seeds. *Lancet.* 1981; 1 (8220 Pt 1): 615.

34. Prete PE. The Mechanism of action of L-canavanine in inducing autoimmune phenomena. *Arthritis & Rheumatism.* 1985; 28 (10): 1985: 1198-1200; Alcocer-VarelaJ, Iglesias L, Liorente L, Alarcon-Segovia D. Effects of L-canavanine on T-cells may explain the induction of systemic lupus erythematosus by alfalfa. *Arthritis & Rheumatism.* 1985; 28 (1): 52-57.

35. Mousa SA. Antithrombotic effects of naturally derived products on coagulation and platelet function. *Methods in Molecular Biology.* 2010; 663: 229-240.

36. Natural Standard: The Authority on Integrative Medicine. Available at: http://www.naturalstandard.com.proxy.libumich.edu/databases/herbssupplements/aloe vera.asp. Accessed December 2011.

37. Morrow DM, Rapaport MJ, Strick RA. Hypersensitivity to aloe. *Arch Dermtol.* 1980; 116: 1064-1065; Ferreira M, Teixeira M, Silva E, et al. Allergic dermatitis to aloe vera. *Contact Dermatitis.* 2007; 57: 278-279.

38. Syed TA, Ahmad Sa Holt AH, et al. Management of psoriasis with aloe vera extract in hydrophilic cream: a placebo-controlled, double-blinded study. *Trop Med Int Health.* 1996; 1: 505-509.

39. Paulsen E, Korsholm L, Brandrup F. A double-blind, placebo-controlled study of a commerical aloe vera gel in the treatment of slight to moderate psoriasis vulgaris. *J Eur Acad Dermatol Vrnereol.* 2005; 19: 326-331.

40. Gennaro AR. *The Science and Practice of Pharmacy.* 19th ed. Philadelphia, PA: Lippinocott Williams & Wilkins Co.; 1996. p. 505.

41. Parfitt K. *Martindale: The Complete Drug Reference.*

42. Ibid.

43. DerMarderosian A. *The Review of Natural Products.* St. Louis, MO:

Facts and Comparison Publishing Group, A Wolters Kluwer Co.; Jan 1999.

44.   Dekker R. Apple juice and the chemical-contact softening of gallstones. *Lancet*. 1999; 354 (9): 18-25.

45.   DerMarderosian A. *The Review of Natural Products*.

46.   Srinivasan K. Role of spices beyond food flavoring: Nutraceuticals with Multiple Health Effects. *Food Rev Int*. 2005; 21 (2): 167-188; Hemla A, Nidhi K, Foods used as ethno-medicine in Jammu. *Ethno-Med*. 2009; 3 (1): 65-68.

47.   Lee CL, Chia-Lin L, Lien-Chai C, et al. Influenza A (H1N1) Antiviral and Cytotoxic Agents from Ferula assa-foetida. *J Nat Prod*. 2009; 72: 1568-1572.

48.   Putt MS, Milleman KR, Ghassemi A, et al. Enhance of plaque removal efficacy by tooth brushing with baking soda dentifrices results of five clinical studies. *J of Clin Dent*. 2008; 19 (4):111-119.

49.   Sobel JD, Faro S, Force RW, et al. VVC: epidemiologic, diagnostic, and therapeutic considerations. *Am J Ostet Gynecol*. 1998; 178: 203-211.

50.   Bozin B, Mimica-Dukic N, Simin N, et al. Characterization of the volatile composition of essential oils of some lamiaceae spices and the antimicrobial and antioxidant activities of the essential oils. *J Agric Food Chem*. 2006; 54 (5): 1822-1828; Chiang LC, Ng LT, Cheng PW, et al. Antiviral activities of extracts and selected pure constituents of Ocimum basilicum. *Clin Exp Pharmacol Physiol*. 2005; 32 (10): 811-816; de Almeida I, Alviano DS, Vieira DP, et al. Antigiardial activity of Ocimum basilicum essential oil. *Parasitol Res*. 2007; 101 (2): 443-452; Manosroi J, Dlumtanom P, Manosroi A. Anti-proliferative activity of essential oil extracted from Thai medicinal plants an KB and P388 cell lines. *Cancer Lett*. 2006; 235 (1): 114-120.

51.   Phasomkusolsil S, Soonwera M. Insect repellent activity of medicinal plant oil against Aedes aegypt (Linn) Anopheles minimus (Theobald) and Culex quinquefasciatus Say based on protection time and biting rate. *Southeast Asia J of Trop Med & Pub Health*. 2010; 41 (4): 831-840.

52.   Gennaro AR. *The Science and Practice of Pharmacy*. 19th ed. Philadelphia, PA: Lippincott Williams & Wilkins Co.; 1996. p. 703.

53. DerMarderosian A. *The Review of Natural Products*. Sep 1992.

54. Tifford GL. *Edible and Medicinal Plants of the West*. 1st ed. Missoula, MT: Mountain Press Publishing Co.; 1997. p. 186.

55. American Pharmaceutical Association. *Handbook of Nonprescription Drugs*. 13th ed. Washington, DC; 2000. p. 316.

56. Dai J, Patel DJ, Jigna D, et al. Characterization of blackberry extract and its anti-proliferative and anti-inflammatory properties. *J of Medicinal Foods*. 2007; 10 (2): 258-265; Seeram NP, Adams LS, Zhang Y, et al. Blackberry, black raspberry, blueberry, cranberry, red raspberry, and strawberry extracts inhibit growth and stimulates apoptosis of human cancer cells in vitro. *J of Agricultural & Food Chem*. 2006; 54 (25): 9329-9339; Ding M, Feng R, Wang SY, et al. Cyanidin-3-glycoside, a natural product derived from blackberry extract exhibits chemopreventive and chemotherapeutic activity. *J of Bio Chem*. 2006; 261 (25): 1759-1769.

57. Gever J. FDA warns of cure-all product based on bleach. Available at: http://www.Medpagetoday.com. Accessed Jul 30, 2010.

58. Stull AJ, Cash KC, Johnson WD, et al. Bioactives in blueberries improve insulin sensitivity in obese, insulin-resistant men and women. *J of Nutrit*. 2010; 40 (10): 1764-1768.

59. Nemis-Nagy E, Scozs-Molnar T, Dunca I, et al. Effects of dietary supplements containing blueberry and sea buckthorn concentrate on antioxidant capacity in type 1 diabetic children. *Acta Physiologica Hungarica*. 2008; 95 (4): 383-393.

60. Neto CC. Cranberry and blueberry: evidence for protection against cancer and vascular diseases. *Molecular Nirtrit and Food Res*. 2007; 51 (6): 652-664.

61. Krikorian R, Shidler MD, Nash TA, el al. Blueberry supplementation improves memory in older adults, *J Agric Food Chem*. 2010; 58 (7): 3996-4000.

62. Hassan S, Shaikh MU, Ali N, et al. Copper sulphate toxicity in a young male complicated by methemoglobinemia, rhabdomyolysis and renal failure. *J Coll Phy Sur Pak*. 2010; 20 (7): 490-491.

63. Gennaro AR. *The Science and Practice of Pharmacy*. p. 1041.

64.   American Pharmaceutical Association. *Handbook of Nonprescription Drugs*. p. 139; Haefner HK. Current evaluation and management of vulvovaginitis.*Clin Obstet Gynecopl.* 1999; 42 (2): 184 195; Sobel JD Vaginitis. *N Eng J Med.* 1997; 337 (26): 1896-1903.

65.   Blumenthal M, Busse WR, Goldberg A, et al., eds. *The Complete German Commission E Monographs: Therapeutic Guide to Herbal Medicines.* Austin, TX: American Botanical Council and Boston Integrative Medicine Communications; 1998. pp. 95-98.

66.   Tieman E, Harris A. Butter in the initial treatment of hot tar burns. *Burns.* 1993; 19 (5): 437-438.

67.   Natural Standard: The Authority on Integrative Medicine. Available at: http://www.naturalstandard.com.proxy.libumich.edu/databases/herbssupplements/calamus.asp. Accessed December 2011.

68.   Taylor JM, Jones WI, Hagan WI, et al. FDA bans calamus as a food or food additive. *Tox and Applied Pcol.* 1967; 10: 405.

69.   Riazuddin S, Malik MM, Nasin A. Mutagenicity testing of some medicinal herbs. *Environ Mol Mutagen.* 1987; 10 (2): 141-148.

70.   Shah AJ, Gilani AH. Blood pressure-lowering and vascular modulator effects of acorus calamus extract are mediated through multiple pathways. *J Cardiovasc Pharmacol.* 2009; 54 (1): 38-46.

71.   Gossel TA. Camphorated oil. *US Pharm.* 1983; 8 (4): 12, 14, 16.

72.   Ragucci KR, Trangmar P, Jefferson GB, et al. Camphor ingestion in a 10-year-old male. *Southern Med J.* 2007; 100 (2): 204-207.

73.   Parfitt, *Martindale: The Complete Drug Reference.* p. 1560.

74.   Medhi B, Kishore K, Singh U, et al. Comparative clinical trials of castor oil and diclofenac sodium in patients with arthritis. *Phytotherapy Res.* 2009; 23 (10): 1469-1473.

75.   McFarlin BL, Gibson MH, O'Rear J, et al. A national survey of herbal preparations used by nurse-midwives for labor stimulation, Review of the literature and recommendations for practice. *J Nur Midwifery.* 1999: 443 (3): 205-216; Azhari S, Pidadeh S, Lotfalizalizadeh M, et al. Evaluation of the effect of castor oil on initiating labor in term pregnancy. *Saudia Med*

J. 2006; 27 (7): 1011-1014.

76. Boel ME, Lee SJ, Rijken MJ, et al. Castor oil for induction of labor not harmful, not helpful. *Astralian & New Zealand J of Obstet & Gyn.* 2009; 49 (5): 499-503.

77. Foster S, Tyler VE. *Tyler's Honest Herbal — A Sensible Guide to the Use of Herbs and Related Remedies.* 4th ed. New York: MJF Books; 1999: 93-95.

78. Graham PH, Browne L, Cox H, et al. Inhalation aromatherapy during radiotherapy results of placebo-controlled double-blind randomized trial. *J of Clin Oncol.* 2003; 21 (12): 2372-2376.

79. Chu YF, Sun J, Wu X, et al. Antioxidant and antiproliferative activity of common vegetable. *J Agri Food Chem.* 2002; 50: 6910-6916; Woods JA, Jewell C, O'Brien NM, et al. Sedanolide, a natural phthalide from celery seed oil: effect on hydrogen peroxide and tert-butyl hydroperoxide-induced toxicity in HepG2 and CaCo-2 human cell lines. *In Vitr Mol Toxicol,* 2001; 14: 233-240.

80. Ljunggren B. Severe phototoxic burn following celery ingestion. *Arch Dermatol.* 1990; 128: 1334-1336; DeLeo VA. Photocontact dermatitis. *Dermal Ther.* 2004; 17: 279-88; Wang L, Sterling B, Berloque DP. Dermatitis induced by "Florida water," *Curtis.* 2002; 70: 29-30; Boffa MJ, Gilmour E, Ead RD. Celery soup causing severe phototoxicity during PUVA therapy. *Br J Dermatol.* 1996; 135: 334; Pulg L, des Moragas JM. Enhancement of PUVA phototoxic effects following celery ingestion; cool broth also can burn. *Arch Dermatol.* 1994; 130: 809-810; Egan CL, Sterling G. Phytophotodermatitis: a visit to Margaritiville, *Curtis.* 1993; 51: 41-42.

81. DerMarderosian A. *The Review of Natural Products.* May 2000.

82. Kato A, Minoshima Y, Yamamoto J, et al. Protective effects of dietary chamomile tea on diabetic complications. *J of Agricul & Food Chem.* 2008; 56 (17): 8206-8211.

83. Mckay DL, Blumberg JB. A review of the bioactivity and potential health benefits of chamomile tea. *Phytotherapy Res.* 2006; 20 (7) 519-530.

84. Taylor JL, Tuttle J, Pramukul T, et al. An outbreak of cholera in Maryland associated with imported commercial frozen fresh coconut milk. *J of Infectious Dis.* 1993; 16 (6): 1330-1335.

85.   Varma SD, Hegde KR, Kovtun S. UV-B-induced damage to the lens: Prevention by caffeine. *J Clin Pharmacol Ther*. 2008; 24 (5): 439-444.

86.   Mikuls TR, Cerhan JR, Criswell LA, et al. Coffee, tea, and caffeine consumption and risk of rheumatoid arthritis results from the Iowa women's health study. *Arthritis & Rheumatism*. 2002; 46 (1): 83-91.

87.   Reed SD, Newton KM, Lacrox AZ, et al. Vaginal, endometrial, and reproductive hormone findings: randomized, placebo-controlled trial of black cohosh, multibotanical herbs and dietary soy for vasomotor symptoms; the herbal alternatives for menopause study. *Menopause*. 2008; 15 (1): 51-58; Ruhlen RL, Haubner J, Tracy JK. Black cohosh does not exert an estrogenic effect on the breast. *Nutrition & Cancer*. 2007; 59 (2): 269-277; Spangler L, Newton KM, Grothaus LC, et al. The effects of black cohosh therapies on lipids, fibrinogen, glucose, and insulin. *Maturitas*. 2007; 57 (2): 195-204.

88.   Geller SE, Studee L. Botanical and dietary supplements for mood and anxiety in menopausal women. *Menopause*. 2007; 14 (3 pt 1); 541-549; Borrelli F, Ernst E. Alternative and complementary therapies for menopause. *Maturitas*. 2010; 66 (4): 333-343; Shams T, Setia MS, Hemmings R, et al. Efficacy of black cohosh-containing preparations on menopausal symptoms: a meta-analysis. *Alternative Therapies in Health & Medicine*. 2010; 16 (1): 36-44; Geller SE, Shulman LP, van Breeman RB, et al. Safety and efficacy of black cohosh and red clove for the management of vasomotor symptoms: a randomized controlled study. *Menopause*. 2009; 16 (6): 1156-1166.

89.   Joy D, Joy J, Duane P. Black cohosh: a cause of abnormal postmenopausal liver function tests. *Climacteric*. 2008; 11 (1): 84-88.

90.   Nasr J, Nafeh H. Influence of black cohosh used by postmenopausal women on total hepatic perfusion and liver function. *Fertility & Sterility*. 2009; 92 (5): 1780-1782.

91.   Roberts H. Safety of herbal medical products in women with breast cancer. *Matuuritas*. 2010; 66: 363-369.

92.   Wu M, Hu Y, Ali Z, et al. Teratogenc effects of blue cohosh (Caulophyllum thalictroides) in Japanese medaka (Oryzias latipes) are probably mediated through GATA2/EDN1 signaling pathway. *Chem Res Toxicol*. 2010; 23 (8): 1405-1408.

93.   McFarlin BL, Gibson MH, O'Rear J, Harman P. A national survey of herbal preparations used by nurse mid-wives for labor stimulation. Review of the literature and recommendations for practice. *J Nurse Midwifery.* 1999; 44 (3): 205-216.

94.   Dugoua JJ, Perri D, Seely D, et al. Safety and efficacy of blue cohosh during pregnancy and lactation. *Can J Clin Pharmacol.* 2008: 15 (1): e66-73.

95.   Tifford GL. *Edible and Medicinal Plants of the West.* p. 38.

96.   Letden JJ, Corn starch, Candida albacans, and diaper rash. *Pediatric Derm.* 1984; 1 (4) 322-325.

97.   Spiller GA, Story JA, Furumoto EJ, et al. Effect of tartaric acid and dietary fiber from sun-dried raisins on colonic function and on bile acid and volatile fatty acid excretion in healthy adults. *Brit J of Nutrition.* 2003; 90 (4): 803-807.

98.   DerMarderosian A. *The Review of Natural Products.* Aug 1998.

99.   Sigstedt SC, Hootten CJ, Callewaert MC, et al. Evaluation of aqueous extracts of Taraxacum officinale on growth and invasion of breast and prostate cancer cells. *Intl J of Oncol.* 2008; 32 (5): 1085-1090.

100. Goksu E, Eken C, Karadeniz O, et al. First report of hypoglycemia secondary to dandelion ingestion. *Amer J of Emrg Med.* 2010; 28 (1): 111. e1-2.

101. Center for Disease Control and Prevention. Respiratory illness associated with inhalation of mushroom spores. Morbidity & Mortality Weekly Report. 1994; 43 (29): 525-526.

102. Tifford GL. *Edible and Medicinal Plants of the West.* p. 124.

103. Chai TJ, Chai TC. Bactericidal activity of cerumen. *Antimicrobial Agents & Chemotherapy.* 1980; 18 (4): 638-641; Stone M. Fulghum, Bactericidal activity of wet cerumen. *Annals of Otology & Laryngology.* 1984; 93 (2 pt 1): 183-186; Megarry S, Pett A, Scarlett A, et al. The activity against yeasts of human cerumen. *J of Laryngology and Otology.* 1988; 102 (8): 671-672.

104. Blitz M, Blitz S, Hughes R, et al. Aerosolized magnesium sulfate for acute asthma: a systemic review. *Chest.* 2005; 128: 337-344.

105. Rowe BH, Bretzlaff JA, Bourdon C, et al. Magnesium sulfate for treating exacerbations of acute asthma in the emergency department. *Cochrane Database Syst Rev*. 2000; (2): CD001490.

106. Parfitt, *Martindale: The Complete Drug Reference*. p. 1157.

107. Salari MH, Amine G, Shirazi MH, et al. Antibacterial effects of eucalyptus globulus leaf extract on pathogenic bacteria isolated from specimens of patients with respiratory track disorders. *Clin Microbiol*. 2006; 12 (2): 194-196.

108. Gobel H, Schmidt G, Soyka D, Effect of peppermint and eucalyptus oil preparations on neurophysiological and experimental algesimetric headache parameters. *Cephalalgia*. 2002; 14 (3): 228-234; Hong C-Z, Shellock FG. Effects of a topically applied counterirritant (Eucalyptmint) on cutaneous blood flow and on skin and muscle temperatures: a placebo-controlled study. *Amer J of Physical Med & Rehab*. 1991; 70 (1): 29-33.

109. Dreisinger N, Zane D, Etwaru K. A poisoning of topical importance. *Ped Emerg Care*. 2006: 22 (12): 827-829.

110. Tabbalis J. Clinical effects and management of eucalyptus oil ingestion in infants and young children. *Med J Aust*. 1995; 163: 177-180.

111. Stoss M, Michels C, Peters E, et al. Prospective cohort trial of Euphrasia single-dose eye drops in conjunctivitis. *J Alter Complement Med*. 2000; 6: 499-508; Mokkapatti R. An experimental double-blind study to evaluate the use of Euphrasia in the prevention of conjunctivitis. *Brit Homeopath J*. 1992; 1: 22-24.

112. Bonakdar RA. *The H.E.R. B. A. L. Guide; Dietary Supplement Resources for the Clinician*. 1st ed. Philadelphia, PA: Wolters Kluwer/ Lippincott Williams & Wilkins; 2010. p. 326.

113. Losso JN, Holiday DL, Findley JW, et al. Fenugreek bread; a treatment for diabetes mellitus. *J of Medicinal Food*. 2009; 12 (5): 1046-1049; Kochhar A, Nagi M. Effect of supplementation of traditional medicinal plants on blood glucose in non-insulin-dependent diabetes: a pilot study. *J of Medicinal Food*; 2005; 8 (4): 545-549; Madar Z, Abel R, Samish S, Arad J. Glucose-lowering effect of fenugreek in non-insulin-dependent diabetes. *European J Clin Nutrit*. 1988; 42 (1): 51-54; Kassaian N, Azadbakht L, Forghani B, et al. Effects of fenugreek seeds on blood glucose and lipid profiles in type 2 diabetes patients. *Intl J for Vitamin & Nutrition Res*. 2009: 79 (1): 34-39.

114. Chevassus A, Gaillard JB, Farret A, et al. A fenugreek seed extract selectivity reduces spontaneous fat intake in overweight subjects. *Europ J Clin Pharmacol*. 2010; 66: 449-455.

115. Serraclara A, Hawkins F, Perez C, et al. Hypoglycemic action of an oral fig-leaf decoction in type 1 diabetic patients. *Diabetes Res Clin Pact*. 1998; 39 (1): 19-22; Perz C, Canal JR, Torres MD. Experimental diabetes treated with ficus carica extract: effect on oxidative stress parameters. *Acta Diabetol*. 2003; 40 (1): 3-8.

116. Basch E, Bent S, Collins J, et al. Flax and flaxseed oil (Linum usitassimum): a review by the National Science Research Collaboration. *J Society for Integrative Oncol*. 2007; 5 (3): 92-105; Pan A, Yu D, Demark-Wahnefried W, et al. Meta-analysis of the effects of flaxseed interventions on blood lipids. *Am J Clin Nutrit*. 2009; 90 (2): 288-297; Demark-Wahnefried W, Polascik TJ. George SI, et al. Flaxseed supplementation (not dietary fat restriction) reduces prostate cancer proliferation rates in men presurgery. *Cancer Epidemiollogy, Biomakers & Prevention*. 2008; 17 (12): 3577-3587; Sturgeon SR, Volpe SL, Puleo E. Effect of flaxseed consumption on urinary levels of estrogen metabolites in postmenopausal women. *Nutrition & Cancer*. 2010; 62 (2): 175-180.

117. Natural Standard: The Authority on Integrative Medicine. Available at: http://www.naturalstandard.com.proxy.libumich.edu/databases/herbssupplements/Garlic.asp. Accessed December 2011.

118. Lissiman E, Bhasale AL, Cohen M. Garlic for the common cold. *Cochrane Database of Systemic Reviews*. 2009; (3): CD006206.

119. DerMarderosian A. *The Review of Natural Products*. May 2000.

120. Bonakdar RA. *The H.E.R. B. A. L. Guide; Dietary Supplement Resources for the Clinician*. pp. 320-321.

121. Rahnama P, Montazeri A, Hassan FH. Effects of Zingiber officinale R. rhizones on pain relief in primary dysmenorrheal: a placebo randomized trial. *BMC Complement Altern Med*. 2012; 12: 92-98.

122. Altman RD, Marcussen KC. Effects of ginger extract on knee pain in patients with osteoarthritis. *Arthritis Rheum*. 2001; 2531-2538.

123. Vuksan V, Sievenpiper JL, Koo VY. American ginseng (Panax quinquefolius) reduces postprandial glycemia in nondiabetic subjects and

subjects with type 2 diabetes. *Achives Int Med*. 2000; 160 (7): 1009-1013; Vuksan V, Stavro MP, Sievepiper JL, et al. Similar postprandial glycemia reductions with escalation of dose and administration of American ginseng in type 2 diabetes. *Diabetes Care*. 2000; 23 (9): 1221-1226.

124. Predy GN, Goel V, Lovlin R. Efficacy of an extract of North American ginseng containing poly-furanosyl-pyranosyl saccharides for prevention of upper respiratory tract infections: a randomized controlled trial. *CMAJ*. 2005; 173 (9): 1043-1049.

125. Pollack A. F.D.A. Approves Drug From Gene-Altered Goats. *New York Times*. February 6, 2009. Available at: http://www.nytimes.com/2009/02/07/business/07goatdrug.html). Accessed August 11, 2011.

126. Trivedi B P. Lab Spins Artificial Spider Silk, Paving the Way to New Materials. National Geographic. January 17, 2002. Avaialble at: http://news.nationalgeographic.com/news/2002/01/0117_020117TVspidermammals.html. Last accessed August 2011.

127. Ingersoll GL, Wasilewski A, Haller M, et al. Effects of concord grape juice on chemotherapy-induced nausea and vomiting: results of a pilot study. *Oncol Nurs Forum*. 2010; 37 (2): 213-221.

128. Kikorian R, Nash TA, Shidler MA, et al. Concord grape juice supplementation improves memory function in older adult with mild cognitive impairment. *Brit J of Nutrition*. 2010; 103 (5): 730-734.

129. Rasmussen D. *American Uprising: The Untold Story of America's Largest Slave Revolt*. 1st ed. New York: Harper Collins Publishers; 2011. p. 31.

130. Rollings-Magnusson S. Flaxseed, goose grease, and gun powder.

131. DerMarderosian A. *The Review of Natural Products*. Nov 1987.

132. Dealleaume L, Tweed B, Neher JO. Do OTC remedies relieve cough in acute URI's?. *J Family Practice*. 2010; 59 (1): 13; Shadkam MN, Mozaffari-Khosravi H, Mozayan MR. A comparison of the effect of honey, dextromethorphan. And dihydramine on nightly cough and sleep quality in children and their parents. *J Alternative & Complimentary Medicine*. 2010; 16 (7): 787-793.

133. Wijesinghe M, Weatherall M, Perrin K, et al. Honey in the treatment of burns: a systemic review and meta-analysis of its efficacy, New Zealand

Med J, 2009; 122 (1295): 47-60; Boukraa L, Sulaiman SA. Honey use in burn management: potentials and limitations. *Forschende Komplementarmedizin.* 2006: 17 (2): 74-80.

134. Foster S, Tyler VE. *Tyler's Honest Herbal.* pp. 217-218.

135. Llewellyn PJ. Billberry, National Center for Complementary and Alternative Medicine. National Institute of Health. July 2010.

136. Parfitt K. *Martindale: The Complete Drug Reference.* p. 1494.

137. Gennaro AR. *The Science and Practice of Pharmacy.* p. 1509.

138. American Pharmaceutical Association. *Handbook of Nonprescription Drugs.* p. 476.

139. Vearrier D, Greenberg MI. Anticholinergic delirium following datura stramonium ingestion: Implications for the internet age. J *Emer Trauma Shock,* 2010; 3 (3): 303-305.

140. Tifford GL. *Edible and Medicinal Plants of the West.* p. 84.

141. DerMarderosian A. *The Review of Natural Products.* Feb 1997.

142. Rollings-Magnusson S. Flaxseed, goose grease, and gun powder. pp. 388-410.

143. Rostami K, Farzaneh E, Abolhassani H. Bilateral deep peroneal nerve paralysis following kerosene self-injection into external hemorrhoids, *Case Reports Medicine.* 2010; 850394.

144. Finnerud CW, Kesler RL, Wiese HF. Ingestion of lard in the treatment of eczema and allied dermatoses. *Archives of Dermat.* 1941; 44 (5): 849-861.

145. Conforti ML. Connors NP, Heisey DM, et al. Evaluation of performance characteristics of the medicinal leeches for the treatment of venous congestion. *Plastic Reconstr Surg.* 2002; 109: 228-235; Riede F, Koenen W, Goerdt S, et al. Medicinal leeches for the treatment of venous congestion and hematoma after plastic reconstruction surgery. *J Disch Dermatol Ges.* 2010; 8 (11): 881-888.

146. DerMarderosian A. *The Review of Natural Products.* April 1999.

128

147. Carper J. *The Food Pharmacy*. New York: Bantam Publishing; 1988. pp. 222-232.

148. Chevallier A. Encyclopedia of Medicinal Plants. New York: DK Publishing Co; 1996. p. 81.

149. Parfitt K. *Martindale: The Complete Drug Reference*. p. 1197.

150. Crean AM, Abdel-Rahman SED, Greenwood JP. A sweet tooth as the root cause of cardiac arrest. *Can J Cardiol*. 2009; 25 (10): e357-e358; Liu JF, Srivatsa A, Kaul V. Black licorice ingestion: yet another confounding agent in patients with melena. *World J Gastrointest Surg*. 2010; 2 (1): 30-31.

151. Elinav E, Chajek-Shaul T. Licorice consumption causing severe hypokalemic paralysis. *Mayo Clin Proc*. 2003; 78: 767-768; Miettinen HE, Pippo K, Hannila-Handelberg T. Licorice hypertension and common variants of gene regulating renal sodium reabsorption. *Ann Med*. 2010; 42: 465-474.

152. Parfitt K. *Martindale: The Complete Drug Reference*. p. 1089.

153. Tifford GL. *Edible and Medicinal Plants of the West*. pp. 96-107.

154. Tunuguntla A, Sullivan MJ. Black strap molasses for the treatment of inflammatory bowel disease-associated anemia. *Southern Med J*. 2004; 97 (8): 794.

155. Lim HC, Poulose V, Tan HH. Acute naphthalene poisoning following the non-accidental ingestion of mothball. *Singapore Med J*. 2009; 50 (8): 298-301; Weintraub E, Gandhi D, Robinson C. Medical complications due to mothball abuse. *Southern Med J*. 2000; 93 (4): 427-429; Siegel E, Wason S. Mothball toxicity. *Ped Clin North America*. 1986; 33 (2): 369-374; Sillery JJ, Lichenstein R, Barrueto F Jr, Teshome G. Hemolytic anemia induced by ingestion of paradichlorobenzene mothballs. *Pediatr Emer Care*. 2009; 25 (4): 252-254.

156. Fine DH, Furgang D, Sinatra K, Charles C, et al. In vivo antimicrobial effectiveness of an essential oil-containing mouth rinse 12 h after a single use and 14 days' use. *J Clin Periodontol*. 2005; 32 (4): 335-340; Charles CA, McGuire JA, Sharma NC, Qagish J. Comparative efficacy of two daily use mouthrinses: randomized clinical trial using an experimental gingivitis model. *Braz Oral Res*. 2011: 25 (4): 338-344; Ross NM, Mankodi Sm, Mostler Kl, et al. Effect of rinsing time on antiplaque-

antigingivitis efficacy of Listerine. *J Clin Periodontol.* 1993; 20 (4): 279-281; Tufekci E, Casagrande ZA, Lindauer Sj, et al. Effectiveness of an essential oil mouthrinse in improving oral health in orthodontic patients. *Angle Orthod.* 2008; 78 (2): 294-298.

157. DerMarderosian A. *The Review of Natural Products.* April 1998.

158. Turker AU, Gurel E. Common mullein (Verbascum rhapsus): recent advances in research. *Phytotherapy Reserch.* 2005; 19 (9): 733-739; McCarthy E, O'Mahony JM. What's in a name? Can mullein weed beat TB where modern drugs are failing?. *Evi Based Complement Alternat Med.* 2011; 2011: 239237.

159. Tifford GL. *Edible and Medicinal Plants of the West.* p. 158.

160. Bhattacharya A, Li Y, Wade KL, et al. Allyl isothiocyanate-rich mustard seed powder inhibits bladder cancer growth and muscle invasion, Carcinogenesis. 2010; 31 (12): 2105-2110.

161. Van Gils C, Cox PA. Ethanobotany of nutmeg in the Spice Islands. *J Ethanopharmacol.* 1994; 42: 117-124; Grover JK, Khandkar S, Vats V, et al. Pharmacological studies of myristica fragrans-antidiarrheal, hypnotic, analgesic and hemodynamic (blood pressure) parameters. *Experimental Clin Pharmacol.* 2002; 24: 675-680; Olajide OA, Ajayl F, Ekhelar AI, et al. Biological effects of myristica fragrans (nutmeg) extract. *Phytother Res.* 1999; 13: 344-345; Narasimhan B, Dhake AS. Antibacterial principles from myristica fragrans seeds. *J Med Food.* 2006; 9: 395-399; Rani P, Khular N. Antimicrobial evaluation of some medicinal plants for their anti-enteric potential against multi-drug resistant Salmonella typhi. *Phytother Res.* 2004; 18: 670-673; Rashid A, Mara DS. Antienterotoxic effect of myristica fragrans (nutmeg) on enterotoxigenic Escherichia coli. *Indian J. Med Res.* 1984; 79: 694-696.

162. Williams EY, West F. The use of nutmeg as a psychotropic: Report of two cases. *J Med Assoc.* 1968; 60 (4): 289-290; Forrester MB. Nutmeg intoxication in Texas. *Human & Experimental Toxicology.* 1998; 24 (11): 563-566; McKenna A, Nordt SP, Ryan J. Acute nutmeg poisoning. *European J Emerg Med.* 2004; 11 (4): 240-241.

163. Cormu C, Remontet L, Noel-Baron F, Nicolas A, et al. A dietary supplement to improve the quality of sleep: a randomized placebo controlled trial. *BMC Complementary & Alternative Med.* 2010; 10: 29.

164. Nothlings U, Murphy SP, Wilkens LR, et al. Flavonols and pancreatic cancer risk: the multiethnic cohort study. *J Epidemiology*. 2007; 166 (8): 924-931.

165. Galeone C, Pelucchi C, Levi F, Negri E, et al. Onion and garlic use and human cancer. *Am J Clin Nutr*. 2006; 84: (5): 1027-1032.

166. Taj Eldin IM, Ahmed EM, Elwahab HMA. Preliminary study of the clinical hypoglycemic effects of allium cepa (red onion) in type and type 2 diabetic patients. *Environ Health Insights*. 2010; 4: 71-77.

167. Kron RE, Litt M, Finnegan LP. Narcotic addition in the newborn differences in behavior generated by methadone and heroin. *International J Clin Pharmacology & Biopharmacy*. 1975; 12 (1-2): 63-69; Sutton LR, Hinderliter SA. Diazepam abuse in pregnant women on methadone maintenance implications for the neonate. *Clin Pediatrics*. 1990; 29 (2): 108-111; Levy M, Spino M. Neonatal withdrawal syndrome: associated drug and pharmacologic management. *Pharmacotherapy*. 1993; 13 (3): 202-211.

168. DerMarderosian A. *The Review of Natural Products*. Feb 1991.

169. Bantle JP, Wylie-Rosett J, Albright AL, et al. Nutrition recommendations and interventions for diabetes: a position statement of the American Diabetes Association. *Diabetes Care*. 2008; 31: S61-S78.

170. Brown HM. Allergenic peatnut oil in milk formulas. *Lancet*. 1991; 338: 1523; Cantani A. Anaphylaxis from peanut oil in infant feedings and medications. *Eur Rev Med Pharmacol Sci*. 1998; 2: 203-206; Lever LR. Peanut and nut allergy, Creams and ointments containing peanut oil may lead to sensitization. *BMJ*. 1996; 313: 299.

171. Fletchers' Arachis Oil Retention Enema (discontinued in the UK - February 2008). Peanut Oil. Avaialble at: http://www.netdoctor.co.uk/meedicines/100001056.html/. Accessed December 2011.

172. Carmichael PG. Pennyroyal metabolites in human poisoning. *Ann Int Med*. 1997; 126 (3): 250-251; Anderson IB, Mullen WH, Meeker JE, et al. Pennyroyal toxicity; measurement of toxic metabolite levels in two cases and a review of the literature. *Ann Int Med*. 1996; 124 (8): 726-734; Bakerink JA, Gospe SM, Dimand RJ, et al. Multiple organ failure after ingestion of pennyroyal oil from herbal tea in two infants. *Pediatrics*. 1992; 98 (5): 944-947.

173. Qutenza: a high dose capsaicin patch. *Pharmacist's Letter/*

Prescriber's Letter. 2010; 26 (5): 260521.

174. Yoshioka M, St-Pierre S, Drapeau V, et al. Effects of red pepper on appetite and energy intake. *Brit J Nurtition.* 1999: 82 (2): 115-123; Bortolotti M, Coccia G, Grossi G, et al. The treatment of functional dyspepsia with red pepper. *Alimentary Pharmacology & Therapeutics.* 2002; 16 (6): 1075-1082; Yoshioka M, Imanaga M, Ueyama H, et al. Maximum tolerable dose of red pepper decrease fat intake independenctly of spicy sensation in the mouth. *Brit J Nutrition.* 2004; 91 (6) 991-995; Satyanarayana MN. Capsaicin and gastric ulcers. *Critical Reviews in Food Science & Nutrition.* 2006; 46 (4): 275-328.

175. Kigler B, Chaudhary S. Peppermint oil. *Am Fam Physician.* 2007; 75: 1027-1030.

176. Melli MS, Rashidi MR, Nokhoodchi A. A randomized trial of peppermint gel, lanolin ointment, and placebo gel to prevent nipple crack in primiparous breast-feeding women. *Med Science Monitor.* 2007; 13 (9): CR406-411.

177. Grigoleit HG, Grigoleit P. Gastrointestinal clinical pharmacology of peppermint oil. *Phytomedicine.* 2005; 12 (8): 607-611; McKay DL, Blumberg JB. A review of the bioactivity and potential health benefits of peppermint tea. *Phytotherapy Research.* 2006; 20 (8): 619-623; Anonymous. Herbal remedies for dyspepsia: peppermint seems effective. *Prescrire International.* 2008; 17 (95): 121-123; Grigoleit HG, Grigoleit P. Peppermint oil in irritable bowel syndrome. *Phytomedicine.* 2005; 12 (8): 601-606.

178. Gennaro AR. *The Science and Practice of Pharmacy.* p. 845.

179. Voeller B, Coulson AH, Bernstein GS. Mineral oil lubricants cause rapid deterioration of latex condoms. *Contraception.* 1989; 39: 95-102.

180. Natural Standard: The Authority on Integrative Medicine. Available at: http://www.naturalstandard.com.proxy.libumich.edu/databases/herbssupplements/Pokeweed.asp. Accessed December 2011.

181. DerMarderosian A. *The Review of Natural Products.* March 1995.

182. Vlachojannis JE, Cameron M, Chrubasik S. Medicinal use of potato-derived products: a systemic review. *Phytotherapy Research.* 2010; 24 (2): 159-162.

183. DerMarderosian A. *The Review of Natural Products.* March 1995.

184. Farajian P, Katsagani M, Zampelas A. Short-term effects of a snack including dried prunes on energy intake and satiety in normal-weight individuals. *Eating Behaviors.* 2010; 11 (3): 201-203.

185. FDA. FDA Drug Safety Communication: New risk management plan and patient medication guide for quinine sulfate. July 8, 2010.

186. US Patent 4261981. Medical compound produced from ragweed. 1976.

187. Simpson M, Parsons M, Greenwood J, et al. Raspberry leaf in pregnancy: its safety and efficacy in labor. *J Midwifery Womens Health.* 2001; 46 (2): 51-59; Hoist L, Haavik S, Nordeng H. Raspberry leaf-should it be recommended to pregnant women?. *Complement Ther Clin Pract.* 2009; 15 (4): 204-208.

188. Tifford GL. *Edible and Medicinal Plants of the West.* p. 12.

189. Lipovac M, Chedraul P, Gruenhut C, et al. Improvement of postmenopausal depressive and anxiety symptoms after treatment with isoflavones derived from red clover extracts. *Maturitas.* 2010; 65 (3): 258-61.

190. Stedman's Medical Dictionary. 21st ed. Baltimore, MD: The Williams & Wilkins Co; 1968. p. 1290.

191. Parfitt K. *Martindale: The Complete Drug Reference.* p. 1212.

192. Akhondzadeh S, Noroozian M, Mohammadi M, et al. Salvia officinalis extract in the treatment of patients with mild to moderate alzheimer's disease: a double blind, randomized and placebo-controlled trial. *J Clin Pharm Ther.* 2003; 28 (1): 53-59. Jinzhou T, Jing S, Xuekai Z, et al. Herbal therapy; a new pathway for the treatment of alzheimer's disease. *Alzheimers Res Ther.* 2010; 2: 30.

193. Hubbert M, Sievers H, Lehnfeld R, Kehrl W. Efficacy and tolerability of a spray with salvia officinalis in the treatment of acute pharyngitis—a randomised, double-blind, placebo-controlled study with adaptive design and interim analysis. *Eur J Med Res.* 2006; 31; 11 (1): 20-26.

194. Bauser D. Daily nasal saline irrigation not recommended for long-term use. American College of Allergy, Asthma, & Immunology. 2009

Annual Scientific Meeting. San Diego, CA.

195. Huang YG, Li Q, Ivanochko G, et al. Novel selective cytotoxicity of wild sarsaparilla rhizome extract. *J Pharm & Pcol.* 2006; 58 (10): 1399-1403; Wang J Li Q Ivanochko G, et al. Anticancer effects of extracts from a North American medicinal plant-wild sarsaparilla. *Anticancer Research.* 2006; 26 (3A): 2157-2164.

196. Parfitt K. *Martindale: The Complete Drug Reference.* p. 1627.

197. DerMarderosian A. *The Review of Natural Products.* July 1998; Yang B, Ni HK. Diagnosis and treatment of spontaneous colonic perforation analysis of 10 cases. *World J of Gastroenterology.* 2008; 14 (28): 4569-4572.

198. Akdogan M, Tamer MN, Cure E, et al. Effect of spearmint teas on androgen levels in women with hirsutism. *Phytotherapy Res.* 2007; 21 (5): 444-447; Grant P. Spearmint herbal tea has significant anti-androgen effects in polycystic ovarian syndrome: a randomized controlled trial. *Phytotherapy Res.* 2010; 24 (2): 186-188.

199. Liu W, Jawerth LM, Sparks FA, et al. Fibrin fibers have extraordinary extensibility and elastically. *Science.* 2006; 313 (5787): 634.

200. Knutson RA, Merbitz LA, Creekmore MA, et al. Use of sugar and povidone-iodine to enhance wound healing five year's experience. *Southern Med J.* 1981; 74 (11): 1329-1335.

201. Parfitt K. *Martindale: The Complete Drug Reference.* p. 1371.

202. Del Rosso JQ, Baum EW. Comprehensive medical management of rosacea: an interim study report and literature review. *J Clin Aesthet Dermatol.* 2008; 1 (1): 20-25; Del Rosso JQ. The use of sodium sulfacetamide 10 %-sulfur 5 % emollient foam in the treatment of acne vulgaris. *J Clin Aesthet.* 2009; 2 (8): 26-29.

203. Natural Standard: The Authority on Integrative Medicine. Available at: http://www.naturalstandard.com.proxy.libumich.edu/databases/herbssupplements/Sunflower Oil.asp. Accessed December 2011.

204. FDA. Final Monograph. 21 CFR 310.502(a): 1997.

205. Gennaro AR. *The Science and Practice of Pharmacy.* 20th ed. Philadelphia, PA: Lippinocott Williams & Wilkins Co.; 2000. pp. 730-732.

206. Nukamal KJ, NacDermott K, Vinson JA. A 6-month randomized pilot study of black tea and cardiovascular risk factors. *Am Heart J.* 2007; 154 (4): 724; Mackenzie T, Leary L, Brooks WB. The effect of an extract of green and black tea on glucose control in adults with type 2 diabetes mellitus: double-blind randomized study. *Metabolism.* 2007; 56 (10): 1340-1344; Trautwein EA, Du Y, Meymen E, et al. Purified black tea theaflavins and theaflavins/catechin supplements did not affect serum lipids in healthy individuals with mildly to moderately elevated cholesterol concentrations. *European J of Nutrition.* 2010; 49 (1): 27-35.

207. Roeder E. Medicinal plants in Europe containing pyrrolizidine alkaloids. *Pharmazie.* 1995; 50 (2): 83-98.

208. Geer RO Jr. Oral manifestations of smokeless tobacco use. *Otolaryngologic Clinics of North America.* 2011; 44 (1): 31-56; Mushtag N, Beebe LA, Thompson DM. Smokeless tobacco and prevalence of cardiovascular disease. *J Okla State Med Assoc.* 2010; 103 (11-12): 539-544; Joshi MS, Verma Y, Gautam AK, et al. Cytogenetic alterations in buccal mucosa cells of chewers if areca nut tobacco. *Archives of Oral Biology.* 2011; 56 (1): 63-67; Gupta R, Gurm H, Bartholomew JR. Smokeless tobacco and cardiovascular risk. *Arch Int Med.* 2004; 164: 1845-1849; Gupta BK, Kaushik A, Panwar RB, et al. Cardiovascular risk factors in tobacco-chewers: a controlled study. *J Assoc Physicians India.* 2007; 55: 27-31.

209. van der Heide F, Wassenaar M, van der Linde LK, et al. Effects of active and passive smoking on crohn's disease and ulcerative colitis in a cohort from a regional hospital. *Eur J Gastroenterol Hepatol.* 2011; 23: 255-261.

210. Dudek W, Wittczek T, Swierczynska-Machura D, et al. Occupational asthma due to turpentine in art painter—case report. *Int J of Occupational Med & Environmental Health.* 2009; 22 (3): 293-295.

211. Barchino-Ortiz L, Cabeza-Martinez R, Lesi-Desil VM, et. al. Allergic contact hobby dermatitis from turpentine. *Allergol Immunopathol.* 2008; 36 (2): 117-119.

212. Khan AJ, Akhtar RP, Fanuqui ZS. Turpentine oil inhalation leading to lung neucrosis and empyema in a toodler. *Ped Emerg Care.* 2006; 22 (5) 355-357.

213. Troulakis G, Tsatsakis AM, Tzatsarakis M, et al. Acute intoxication and recovery following massive turpentine ingestion: clinical and toxicological data. *Vet Hum Toxicol.* 1997; 39 (3): 155-157.

214. Brunton PA, Hussain A. The erosive effect of herbal tea on dental enamel. *J Dent*. 2001; 29: 517-520.

215. Garcia AF, Cabal C, Losada J, et al. In vivo action of Vanillin on delay time determined by magnetic relaxation. *Hemoglobin*. 2005; 29: 181-187.

216. Paul I. Vapor Rub, petrolatum, and no treatment for children with nocturnal cough and cold symptoms. *Pediatrics*. 2010; 10: 1601.

217. Abanses JC. Vick's Vapor Rub induces mucin secretion, decreases ciliary beat frequency and increases tracheal mucus transport in the ferret trachea. *Chest*. 2009; 135: 143-148.

218. Nolles K, Pratt M. Contact dermatitis to Vick's Vapor Rub. *Dermatitis*. 2010; 21 (3): 167-169.

219. *J Am Board Fam Med*. January-February 2011; 24 (1): 69-74.

220. Parfitt K. *Martindale: The Complete Drug Reference*. p. 1541.

221. Birsa LM, Verity PG, Lee RF. Evaluation of the effects of various chemicals on discharge of and pain caused by jellyfish nematocysts, Comp *Biochem Physiol C Toxicol Pharmacol*. 2010; 151 (4): 426-430.

222. Devore EE, Grodstein F, van Rooji FJ. Dietary antioxidants and long-term risk of dementia. *Arch of Neurology*. 2010; 67 (7): 819-825.

223. Klein EL, Thompson IM, Tangen CM, et al. Vitamin E and the risk of prostate cancer: Results of the selenium and vitamin E cancer prevention trial (SELECT). *JAMA*. 2011; 306 (14): 1549-1556.

224. Banel DK, Hu FB. Effects of walnut consumption on blood lipids and other cardiovascular risk factors: a meta-analysis and systemic review. *Amer J of Clin Nutrition*. 2009; 90 (1): 56-63.

225. Patil B. Watermelon may have Viagra-effect. *Science Daily*. July 1, 2008.

226. Natural Standard: The Authority on Integrative Medicine. Available at: http://www.naturalstandard.com.proxy.libumich.edu/databases/ herbssupplements/Witch hazel.asp. Accessed December 2011.

About the Authors

Eddie L. Boyd earned a doctor of pharmacy degree in 1970 from the University of California, School of Pharmacy at the Medical Center in San Francisco. Upon graduation, Boyd remained at the School of Pharmacy to teach for a year. In 1971 he accepted a position as an assistant professor at the University of Michigan College of Pharmacy. Boyd remained on the faculty for twenty years, and while there, implemented the teaching of the first nonprescription drug courses, the first course on herbal products, and the first community pharmacy clerkship program. While on the faculty of the University of Michigan, he also earned a masters degree in statistics and research methodology from the University of Michigan, School of Public Health. In 1991, he accepted a position as Associate Dean and Director of Research at the College of Pharmacy at Xavier University of Louisiana. In 1993 he returned to the University Michigan College of Pharmacy faculty until his retirement in 2003.

Boyd has published numerous articles in pharmacy, medical education, and scientific journals, as well as chapters in pharmacy textbooks. He has served as an expert witness in nearly one hundred drug cases for the Attorney General in the State of Michigan, the US Attorney's Office, and with private attorneys. The Drug Enforcement Administration United States Department of Justice presented Boyd with a Certificate of Appreciation for Outstanding Contributions in the Field of Drug Law Enforcement.

Over the course of his career, Boyd has received numerous awards and honors, including the School of Pharmacy of San Francisco's Bowl of Hygiea award for academic merit. Boyd was the first and is still the only African American student to ever receive the award. He has worked with the administrators and faculties at both the School of Pharmacy at the University of California and College of Pharmacy at the University of Michigan to establish minority recruitment and retention programs that have led to the recruitment and graduation of approximately one hundred and fifty African American students from those programs.

Today, Boyd resides in Destrehan, Louisiana, where he discusses the use of home remedies by African Americans at Destrehan Plantation all day, every other Friday, to an audience of tourists from all over the world.

Leslie A. Shimp earned her bachelor degree in pharmacy and her doctor of pharmacy degree from the University of Michigan College of Pharmacy in Ann Arbor, Michigan. In 1976 she completed a clinical pharmacy residency program at Buffalo General Hospital in Buffalo, New York. That same year she joined the University of Michigan College of Pharmacy faculty. While teaching at the university she also completed a Specialist in Aging Certificate Program at the University of Michigan Institute of Gerontology and a master's program in clinical research design and statistical analysis at the University of Michigan School of Public Health.

Currently she is a professor of pharmacy at the University of Michigan College of Pharmacy and an Ambulatory Care Clinical Pharmacist with the University of Michigan Health System.

Shimp has advocated strongly for the education of pharmacists in herbal and complementary and alternative medicine (CAM). She helped to develop educational coursework for the University of Michigan College of Pharmacy curriculum on these topics. In 2002-2003 she completed the Faculty Scholars Program in Integrative Healthcare offered by the Complementary and Alternative Medicine Research Center at the University of Michigan. She used this education to further develop CAM teaching within the doctor of pharmacy program at the University of Michigan College of Pharmacy. When she practiced as a clinical pharmacist with the integrative medicine program within the University of Michigan Department of Family Medicine she also developed a student clerkship in integrative pharmacy for pharmacy students.

Shimp has produced about ninety publications, including multiple articles in the pharmacy and medical literature, book chapters, and books. She has been recognized three times for achievements in pharmacy practice. The first award was presented to her in 2006 for an innovative practice established in integrative medicine. Two other awards were received in 2011 from the Michigan Pharmacists Association and the American Society of Health- System Pharmacists to recognize the Patient-Centered Medical Home practice model created and implemented by the University of Michigan Ambulatory Care Clinical Pharmacists.

Shimp continues to be interested in herbal and CAM therapies. She is currently part of a group working to establish an evidence-based medicinal plants garden at the University of Michigan Matthaei Botanical Gardens. She resides in Ann Arbor, Michigan.

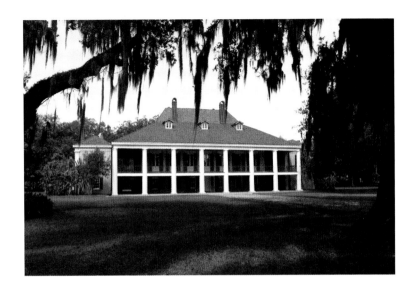

At Destrehan Plantation, a historic house museum in Destrehan, Louisiana, we take pride in telling the unique history of the area. The life of all the inhabitants of the plantation, including slaves, is a vital part of our tour. It is also important that the information provided is as accurate and complete as possible. This book regarding the use of home remedies and herbs passed down from slaves and early generations of African Americans is a wonderful resource and connects the ingenuity of the past to present-day practices.

Nancy J. Robert
Executive Director
Destrehan Plantation, Louisiana